HEADLANDS

HEADLANDS

New Stories of Anxiety

Edited and with an Introduction

by NAOMI ARNOLD

Victoria University Press

TE WHARE WĀNANGA O TE ŪPOKO O TE IKA A MĀUI
VICTORIA
UNIVERSITY OF WELLINGTON

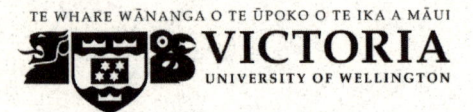

VICTORIA UNIVERSITY PRESS
Victoria University of Wellington
PO Box 600 Wellington
vup.victoria.ac.nz

Copyright © 2018 Naomi Arnold and contributors
First published 2018

This book is copyright. Apart from
any fair dealing for the purpose of private study,
research, criticism or review, as permitted under the
Copyright Act, no part may be reproduced by any
process without the permission of the publishers.
The moral right of the authors has been asserted.

ISBN 9781776561896

A catalogue record for this book is available from the
National Library of New Zealand.

Printed in China by 1010 International Print Group

CONTENTS

Introduction   9
NAOMI ARNOLD

Arise and Pass Away   17
DANYL McLAUCHLAN

Lucky to Be Here   27
REBECCA PRIESTLEY

Water Wings   43
SARAH LIN WILSON

What Happens   49
ZION TAUAMITI

Not Standing Upright There   55
PAUL STANLEY WARD

The Beginning   64
AIMIE CRONIN

In a Scorched Room   70
MICHELLE LANGSTONE

Dream Selves   77
KIRSTEN McDOUGALL

On Citalopram   86
ANTHONY BYRT

Fake It Till You Make It EAMONN MARRA	94
It Needs to Start Early An Interview with RIKI GOOCH	100
Voices DONNA McLEOD	110
Showing Up HINEMOANA BAKER	115
Naming BONNIE ETHERINGTON	125
Mrs Housewife HOLLY WALKER	131
The Curse Machine KATE KENNEDY	138
Worry People MADELINE REID	147
Scared to Death KERRY SUNDERLAND	155
Anxiety in the Body ROSEMARY MANNERING	164
Earnest PSA SUSAN STRONGMAN	171

Side Effects — 176
PAULA HARRIS

Writing from a Dark Place — 187
LEE MURRAY

Moving Earth — 195
SELINA TUSITALA MARSH

Sit in the Fire — 202
JESS McALLEN

The Midst — 209
ALLAN DREW

My Geography — 215
YVETTE WALKER

A Short History of Unease — 221
D.A. GLYNN

Micronutrients and Mental Health — 230
MEREDITH BLAMPIED and JULIA RUCKLIDGE

Ghost Knife — 242
ASHLEIGH YOUNG

Mountain View Road — 255
MIKEY DAM

As Fresh as They Come — 261
TUSIATA AVIA

Contributors — 267

Introduction

Naomi Arnold

Recently, while travelling, I fell into conversation with an older man about this book, and we got talking about anxiety. 'Oh, I had a very anxious period in my youth,' he said, and told me of the time in his mid 20s when he'd started a new job. He worried every day that he was failing, drowning in the unfamiliar environment, afraid of making a mistake. 'But I just wrote myself a list every day before I left work and made sure I ticked it off in the morning,' he said. 'It's about setting priorities. That's how you get over nerves.'

I have heard many versions of this story in the nearly two years since this book was first conceived, and I'll say here what I said in response: Nope. That is not anxiety. If you haven't experienced this illness it can be difficult to understand it, and thus it can be hard to have empathy for how it manifests. We say stuff like: Don't worry, just breathe, chill out, have you tried yoga?

You might have felt tense and worried since you were a small child, or maybe your anxiety developed from trauma, cumulative stress, a change in relationships, brain chemistry, gut biota. But what people with anxiety share is a sense of fear, overwhelming to the point that it interferes in their daily lives and begins to drive every decision.

Clinical anxiety is chronic, crushing panic. Sometimes you can function fine with a faint residual fluttering and a few deep breaths. Other times, it grows until it takes over your mind, your gut, your heart, your breath, your limbs and everything in your life, until your entire being feels reduced to the nub of your earliest brain, the one that pumps adrenaline through your system, puts everything on red alert, shuts down all your body systems, and makes every cell scream: You are in danger. FIGHT. *RUN.*

Bringing this collection together was a delicate task. There's still a stigma in talking about mental health. We—Holly Hunter, Ashleigh Young, Kirsten McDougall and I—approached writers who we knew had anxiety, writers we suspected had anxiety, people with anxiety who we suspected could write, and people with anxiety who didn't necessarily want to write something but had an important story to tell.

In the end, we got yeses from around a hundred people. The next part was more difficult: prompting and encouraging those writers, like all editors do, without making life worse for them. People with anxiety sometimes say yes when they probably should have said no; they are often busy perfectionists, high achievers who put pressure on themselves. But deadlines and publishers can't be put off forever. As we got to the final stages of the book, life—and anxiety—got in the way for many of them. I heard dozens of reasons for why writers felt unable to finish their contributions, or suddenly felt unsafe in revealing so much of themselves, or struggled with a new personal crisis. Some simply dropped off the face of the Earth. 'Attempting to write about life with anxiety (and everything else) caused me massive anxiety and I had to step back from everything for a bit,' was one response, echoed by many. I began to feel the quickening throbs of their hearts between the lines of their emails.

It became clear that many people are suffering intensely, and often without much understanding of what they're going through. Some told me, 'I've never really articulated this before,' and 'I don't think I'm at the stage of my illness where I know how to talk about it,' and, 'This is new and I don't know what it is yet.'

It also became clear that, despite the overall perception of mental illness in the public eye, the stigma is heavier for some than for others. In selecting the essays for this book, we naturally wanted to hear from as diverse a spread of voices as possible. After a year and a half of searching, phoning, emailing and a massive response to a Twitter call-out, *Headlands* still has some gaps in representation. As I made inquiries, I heard frequently that it's easier and more acceptable for Pākehā not only to access care for mental illness, but to be diagnosed with it in the first place—and that's before considering the type, appropriateness and quality of the available healthcare.

Although it's hard for all, anxiety is more acceptable in some worlds. It's still easier for some to talk about it, to be accepted by friends, family and workplaces, to have a public meltdown and to navigate our flawed mental-health system. White women, for example, can look to plenty of figures in popular media who model what used to be called neuroticism: Ally McBeal, Carrie Bradshaw, Elaine Benes, Liz Lemon, manic pixie dream girls. There are white women columnists in major newspapers who regularly write about their mental-health struggles, including Australian Sarah Wilson (a different Sarah Wilson from the one included in this collection), who recently wrote a revealing memoir about the depths and textures of her anxiety that became a *New York Times* bestseller.

Without generalising, I think it's important to point out that Māori, Pacific Island and Asian communities in New Zealand do not walk the same path with mental illness as Pākehā do, and that a lot of Pākehā, as well as our medical models of healing, don't recognise that. Research shows that these groups are the most likely to experience mental illness, and also the most unlikely to find help for it. As one person I contacted put it, non-Pākehā are less likely to end up in a situation where they'll see someone who'll diagnose them. 'Nobody I know except my Pākehā friends have seen a psychiatrist and are on meds,' she said.

We need to understand how mental illness affects different communities in different ways, and how best to get different people the different kinds of help they need. Sometimes, no matter how many ads and programmes urge you to 'reach out', you might not even recognise that you *have* anxiety, let alone be able to ask for help. The ability of people to reach out successfully is also about the rest of the population reaching in: learning, listening, accepting and building accessible and appropriate pathways, whether that's in the workplace, family, community or health systems.

The essays in this book display anxiety in all its forms: weird, funny, ridiculous, sobering, devastating. They examine anxiety in rich, illuminating detail, discussing how anxiety sits in society, along with treatment plans, methods of coping—and revelations of barely coping, when simply being in the world is too much.

Though we wanted *Headlands* to focus on being anxious and looking out, some of the pieces collected here discuss professionals looking *in* on anxiety. Physiotherapist Rosemary Mannering discusses how anxiety manifests in the body; Zion Tauamiti shares his experience as a suicide prevention officer working with anxious young people; and University of Canterbury clinical psychologists Meredith Blampied and Julia Rucklidge discuss their work with micronutrients as an alternative approach to traditional psychiatric medication.

But this isn't a book of solutions—it is proudly one of problems. Some of those in our collection talk about what they've found useful, but all admit how much of a mess they feel sometimes, and how that's affected their relationships with family and friends. People can lose their patience with those who have anxiety, or any mental illness. We might like to think we're all supportive and helpful, but it takes a great deal of empathy and experience to stick with someone who's exhibiting all the frustrating and confusing behaviour that comes with mental illness.

From an outsider's perspective, what helps people with anxiety is letting them talk, giving them time, offering friendship and forgiveness, a place of safety, understanding and respect for their autonomy. That's where this book comes in. Anxiety can be difficult and troubling for those outside it. Its sufferers can seem flaky, isolate themselves, have 'inappropriately emotional' reactions. They might not sleep; they might fear rejection and lash out. Their friends might drift away, confused by their behaviour. They're both hamstrung by fear and chronically conscientious and sensitive. They might also be incredibly frustrated when any emotion or reaction they do have is dismissed because of their anxiety. Don't ask an anxious person, 'Have you tried yoga/veganism/meditation/interval training?' They know. They have tried everything, and yet here they are.

If you have anxiety, the voices in this collection offer reassurance and validation. They know what it's like to be unable to pull the keys from the car ignition and go to a party, as Hinemoana Baker experiences. To be a Māori woman and thus not permitted to fall apart, as Donna McLeod writes in a mesmerising piece, because you're the one holding it all together. To dread your friends' reactions to your panic attack, as Susan Strongman reveals in 'Earnest PSA'. To find yourself inside a mental health secure unit, as Paula Harris describes in a bracing essay on the source of her anxiety. To suddenly discover, as Tusiata Avia has, that many of your health symptoms are related to anxiety, and to try to figure out what on earth to do now.

The voices here know what it's like to struggle for breath, to curl up on the cool bathroom floor, to avoid going out. To not know how to relax, like others can. To sit in the office bathroom and try to do your breathing. To spend night after night listening to meditation apps, only to lose hours of darkness to a thrashing heart and awake at three in the morning gasping for breath. To stay awake until dawn—and then get up anyway, facing the world with sand in your eyes and a fist punching your gut.

The writers in this collection are not alone. In 2017, one in five New Zealanders sought help for a diagnosed mood or anxiety disorder—the same percentage of the population that texts while driving, lies about the number of people they've had sex with, sees no problem with accessing social networks at the office, and are still working over 65. But the real figures will be even higher than that, and they're growing. Ministry of Health figures for the same year reveal that nearly 20 percent of people were diagnosed with a mood and anxiety disorder, up from 12.7 percent in 2007. Thousands more will have stayed silent. This book is for you.

HEADLANDS

Arise and Pass Away

Danyl McLauchlan

I never wanted to be mindful. All I wanted was to get some sleep. For weeks I'd been waking in the middle of the night. Sometimes I lay there thinking obsessively about work; other nights I had fragments of songs looping in my head. I'd read somewhere that our brains recycle thoughts or pieces of music because it saves energy and one night I lay awake thinking 'I'm thinking this thought to save energy' over and over again until dawn.

Another night I pulled on some track pants and a sweater and went for a walk. It was about three o'clock. Very calm. The sky glowed with stars. I could hear the hum of the powerlines and the sound of the stream at the bottom of the hill. I could also hear music. A choir. I couldn't make out the tune. Possibly a hymn? My first thought was: someone is playing their stereo way too loud. But then the music stopped and I heard a man's voice and a woman's laughter and the song began again from the beginning, a little faster and stronger, and I realised the music came from an actual choir of people somewhere nearby. What kind of choir practised at three in the morning?

It sounded as if it came from the school. I crossed the road, treading carefully in my bare feet, and walked up the driveway. Whoever they were, I thought, it would be nice to stand at the back of the hall and listen to a big group of people singing together. It might calm my troubled brain and help me sleep. But when I got to the top of the driveway all the buildings were dark. There was no one there.

There was wind in the trees and I had to wait for it to die down to get a fix on the sound. Then the singing returned, very clearly: a strong, joyous chant. It came from further down the valley. Which made sense: there was a church over there. The hills must have complicated the acoustics. I set off in that direction, breaking into a light jog.

'An auditory hallucination,' my doctor said the next morning. 'Probably tied to the sleep deprivation.'

'Probably tied? You think?' I slouched in a chair, still dressed in the same tracksuit pants I'd worn the night before although they were now splattered with mud. I'd tried to follow the music through the unlit tracks of the town green belt at the bottom of the valley before finally figuring out that it wasn't real and returning home. I'd been awake ever since.

I squinted at my doctor. His office looked out over Wellington Harbour. It was a bright autumn day and the light from the sea and clouds turned the windows into blinding squares of silver and white light. The doctor was a vague, shimmering figure in the foreground. All I wanted was to lie down in a dark room and close my eyes.

'Why can't I sleep?' I demanded. 'Why is this happening? I don't drink. I don't take drugs. I've cut out caffeine. I drink peppermint tea, like an animal. And now this. I can't be wandering around my neighbourhood in the middle of the night, hallucinating. It's completely inappropriate.'

'You say the insomnia started about a month ago,' he said, looking from his notes to a calendar on his computer. 'Which takes us back to daylight saving. Maybe that was the trigger? Sometimes the sleep cycles get confused. We'll try you on sleeping pills for a couple of days, then you can try and sleep without them and see how you go.'

'What if that doesn't work?' I knew there was a link between insomnia and depression, that the conditions amplified each other; I worried that if I didn't treat the insomnia I'd get depressed again, or that I was already depressed and that was causing the insomnia. If I had to go back on antidepressants then I would, but they made me gain weight, made me feel sedated, and coming off them was pure misery, so I'd really rather not. I explained all this in a long, rambling speech; my doctor listened, shimmering patiently, then said, 'From what I'm hearing I think you're suffering from anxiety, not depression.'

'Great. Anxiety. Brilliant.'

'But the medications are pretty much the same.'

'Oh.'

The sleeping pills gave me six hours of deep, dreamless sleep and a metallic taste in my mouth. After three days I went back to unmedicated sleep and woke in the middle of the night. Same thing the next night. The following morning I went to the pharmacy and filled my prescription for nortriptyline, a tricyclic antidepressant with a side effect of sedation. The box came with bright yellow stickers advising me not to operate heavy machinery or expose myself to bright sunlight.

The nortriptyline worked. Overnight. But I wasn't happy to be on it and immediately started plotting to discontinue. 'You should try meditating,' my wife suggested. 'That's supposed to be good for anxiety.'

She'd read this on Facebook but it turned out to be true. A search through the literature turned up a 2010 meta-analysis published in the *Journal of Consulting and Clinical Psychology*. 'Based on 39 studies totalling 1,140 participants receiving mindfulness-based therapy for a range of conditions, including cancer, generalized anxiety disorder, depression, and other psychiatric or medical conditions', the study found that meditation had 'a large, robust effect size for improving anxiety and mood disorders'.[1] And so, reassuring myself that mindfulness was an effective clinical treatment and not pointless New-Age bullshit, I went along to a Buddhist

---

1   S.G. Hofman, A.T. Sawyer, A.A. Witt and D. Oh, 'The Effect of Mindfulness-based Therapy on Anxiety and Depression: A Meta-analytic Review', *Journal of Consulting and Clinical Psychology* 27, no. 2 (April 2010), 169.

meditation evening. It was held in a church (the church noticeboard was filled with flyers advertising yoga evenings and T'ai Chi classes, and I felt a bit sorry for contemporary Christianity: it's not as if temples in India are filled with people flocking to learn the mystical secrets of Protestantism, or how to illuminate manuscripts).

The evening was not a success. At least not for me. A monk appeared, shaved head, saffron robes and all, and talked to us about universal joy and meaningful compassion. Then we meditated on these subjects. I sat in my chair in the warm room and tried to explore joy and compassion but my mind wandered to other things. I felt bored. I spent most of the session thinking about how weird it was to sit in silence with my eyes shut in a room full of strangers. I went home feeling unenlightened and unimpressed. I decided that meditation was not for me.

A week after that, an interview with Robert Wright showed up in my social media feed. Wright was an author and academic: he'd written books about game theory and evolutionary psychology, and his new book was called *Why Buddhism Is True*. He didn't mean it was true in the metaphysical sense, he explained in the interview, or that any other religions were false; rather, he argued that its 'diagnosis of the human predicament' was correct.[2] He talked about the dopaminergic pathways in our brains: clusters of neurons that make us feel good whenever we engage in behaviour that our genes want to encourage, like eating, sex, acquiring material things, increasing our social status. The reward is fleeting, though, so we engage in the same behaviour over and over again, compulsively, chasing ever-decreasing bursts of pleasure, feeling less and less fulfilled. We're not designed by natural selection to be happy, Wright

---

[2] Robert Wright, *Why Buddhism Is True* (New York, NY: Simon & Schuster, 2017), 14.

was saying. But meditation, he claimed, allowed us to escape the hedonic treadmill.

Wright spoke my language. Dopamine. Natural selection. Neuroscience. Let the monks keep their compassion and universal joy. His book was a collection of theoretical essays but Amazon's algorithm served me up a number of books related to the Secular Buddhist movement containing practical instructions on how to meditate. I ordered *The Mind Illuminated* by John Yates, a former lecturer in physiology and neuroscience who discovered Buddhism, changed his name to 'Culadasa'—a Pali word meaning 'lesser servant'—retired from academia, and moved to an old Apache stronghold in the southeastern Arizona wilderness to live a contemplative life.

I meditated every day while waiting for the book to arrive, working off half-remembered instructions from the monk and a general sense that meditation was basically just sitting there and doing nothing, and how hard could that be? I sat every evening, letting my mind wander until I felt drowsy and a sleepy contentment came over me. I found it relaxing. Undemanding. Pleasant. It didn't do much for my overall mood, though. After two weeks of this, Culadasa's book arrived and told me that I'd been doing everything wrong.

The goal of meditation, Culadasa explained, is to improve your attention and awareness, the cognitive faculties with which we perceive—well—everything. At least, that's the goal at first. He defines attention as sustained concentration and awareness as the mind's perception of things outside the scope of concentration. Your attention is on the words you're reading right now; your awareness is capturing the sounds in the background. Attention is developed by concentrating on the sensation of the breath at the nose, awareness by monitoring the thoughts that arise while you're doing this.[3]

---

3 Culadasa, *The Mind Illuminated* (New York, NY: Touchstone Books, 2015), 19–41.

Like most people who begin to meditate, I quickly learned that my ability to pay sustained attention to anything was non-existent; after a few seconds of concentrating on the breath my mind wandered, until I realised I was distracted, then refocussed, and then it wandered again. The book has many tips and exercises for overcoming mind-wandering. Follow them diligently and you will be able to focus on the breath, for a little while, until your brain assumes you're trying to fall asleep and you become drowsy and start to experience strange thoughts and see hypnagogic patterns in the blackness of your eyelids and eventually drift off.

The book employs an old Buddhist metaphor: the mind is like a baby elephant. If you tether it to the ground it will run around and strain at the leash, and then it will fall asleep. There are more tips and exercises to counter this sleepiness, which the book refers to as 'strong dullness'. After strong dullness, you run into physical discomforts: pain in your knees, your back, itches in your face. More exercises. Then, once you've overcome mind-wandering, physical discomfort and strong dullness, you have to contend with 'subtle dullness': the awake-but-still-not-alert condition in which we spend most of our lives. There are yet more exercises for this and they, like all the other exercises, are rather boring. I wouldn't bother with them for even a week, let alone the months I'd been performing them, if they didn't have the baffling but overwhelming side effects of making me feel more focussed, less anxious; peaceful and calm.

'So this is what it's like to be sane and happy,' I marvelled to my wife. We were supermarket shopping and I beamed at the products in the pets aisle—the automated feeders, the plastic dog bones, the worming tablets—which all glowed with a soft inner light.

'I'm glad you're happy,' she replied, choosing her words rather carefully, I thought. But I was happy. There are a number of online communities based around *The Mind Illuminated* and its teachings, and in a somewhat eerie testimony to the efficacy of the system the commentators in these communities are universally friendly and compassionate towards each other, in stark contrast to every other internet community I've seen. The message boards are filled with people suffering from depression, anxiety and other mood disorders who have discovered the book and meditated their way to happiness. But they are also filled with more experienced meditators warning that meditation is a journey, that parts of that journey could be very challenging, that everyone experiences setbacks and disappointments and that you should definitely not abruptly discontinue your medication based on initial success. I decided to stay on the nortriptyline. For now.

If you run every day you become physically fitter: meditating every day seemed to make me psychologically and emotionally fitter. I still felt stress and disappointment and frustration and rage, but the situations that provoked these responses seemed to have the volume turned down, and my mind didn't cultivate self-loathing or rage-inducing thoughts the way it used to. They came and then faded away. People talked a lot of nonsense about meditation, I decided. They made it seem more complicated and mystical than it actually was. Really it was just a form of exercise that made you psychologically more robust. That was all.

The French neuroscientist Stanislas Dehaene once wrote about what we'd see if we could look through our eyes directly, without all the mind's real-time image processing:

> We never see the world as our retina sees it. In fact, it would be a pretty horrible sight: a highly distorted set of light and dark pixels, blown up toward the center of the retina, masked by blood vessels, with a massive hole at the location of the 'blind spot' where cables leave for the brain; the image would

constantly blur and change as our gaze moved around. What we see, instead, is a three-dimensional scene, corrected for retinal defects, mended at the blind spot, stabilized for our eye and head movements, and massively reinterpreted based on our previous experience of similar visual scenes. All these operations unfold unconsciously—although many of them are so complicated that they resist computer-modeling. For instance, our visual system detects the presence of shadows in the image and removes them. At a glance, our brain unconsciously infers the sources of lights and deduces the shape, opacity, reflectance, and luminance of the objects.[4]

I thought about Dehaene's writing when I had an odd, unsettling experience. I'd been meditating for about three months, and one morning I discovered that if I concentrated on the sensations of the breath at my nose for long enough, the feeling of continuous conscious sensation—the feeling you'll get right now if you focus on your own breathing—decohered, breaking down into a series of discrete, meaningless vibrations. It was a little like saying the same word over and over again until it lost its meaning, only the decoherence was with my thoughts themselves. After I ended the session I figured that I'd encountered the raw signal from my sensory system, without any of the usual layering or processing.

It's one thing to understand in theory that your thoughts consist of electrochemical constructs in the brain, but the direct experience of this was surprisingly upsetting. I spent the rest of the day thinking of my body as a kind of robot made of meat designed to transport my brain around and supply it with data and energy. Which of course it is, but I felt that wasn't a healthy way to think about it. And I thought about Yeats' phrase

---

[4] Stanislas Dehaene, *Consciousness and the Brain: Deciphering How the Brain Codes Our Thoughts* (New York, NY: Viking, 2014), 60.

that he was a soul 'fastened to the body of a dying animal'. Over the next week I felt odd pulses of energy fluctuating around my body. I still felt happy, but I worried that my depression or anxiety or whatever the hell it is was ruining my meditation.

I hadn't bothered to finish *The Mind Illuminated*. It's a big book; I'm a busy guy. I'd read the basic stuff about how to meditate and about all of the hindrances I'd encountered and how to overcome them, but that was it. Now I read ahead and discovered that this decoherence and solipsism, the weird energy fluctuations, the intimations of death, were all normal, even desirable.

Modern philosophy in the Western tradition starts with Descartes' famous dictum that we think, therefore we are. We can doubt everything except that the individual self exists, and is thinking, and most of us are happy to go along with that. But Nietzsche, writing in the late 19th century, disputed Descartes. After observing his own mind he noted that *something* thinks, but he had little control over it: he merely observed its thoughts. The Buddhists came to a similar but deeper conclusion two and a half thousand years earlier. What we call the mind, they argue, is really a large aggregation of sub-minds all performing separate tasks that we are mostly unaware of, and our consciousness is just a kind of clearing house or whiteboard for the sub-minds to share information and collaborate on decision-making. There is no 'self', they tell us. The sub-minds share their brief, fleeting impressions and these arise and pass away. Culadasa points out that this model is almost identical to the modular theory of mind currently popular in cognitive psychology.

The importance of mindfulness in this tradition is not to feel relaxed as we drift around the supermarket, although that may be a pleasurable side effect. The goal of the practice is to train the mind to realise the three characteristics that the Buddhists claim are central to existence: the impermanence of the material world, the centrality of suffering and the non-existence of the self. There's no point in understanding any of these things intellectually, the Buddha claimed. You have to meditate and experience them directly, and these experiences can be transformational and, eventually, he claimed, release you from unhappiness. But they can also be troubling—the final appendix in *The Mind Illuminated* is ominously titled 'The Dark Night of the Soul'. The peace and equanimity you gain from mindfulness meditation is designed to help you cope with the insight that you don't really exist, and that everything else you know about reality is allegedly wrong.

I feel a little suckered by mindfulness. I still meditate every day. I highly recommend it over sleeplessness and anxiety and wandering around in the dark, hallucinating. I manage not to think about impermanence or non-existence, much. But every now and then I have another unsettling experience that reminds me that I'm messing around with my central nervous system in ways that aren't documented in the owner's manual. It reminds me that in the eyes of Buddhists and neuroscientists I'm not a sometimes sleepless, sometimes anxious, sometimes medicated, sometimes depressed, often bewildered middle-aged man, that I'm not even a person at all, but rather a cacophony of neural algorithms, a flood of impressions and vibrations no more individual and enduring than a fire started at night that burns until daybreak.

Lucky to Be Here

Rebecca Priestley

'Scott Base, Scott Base, this is K001-Bravo, on 5400, over.'

Richard, sitting near the entrance to the tent, is speaking into the mic of the high-frequency radio. After a minute of static, as the radio waves bounce between the ice and the ionosphere on the way from Friis Hills to Ross Island and back, there's a reply. 'K001-Bravo, this is Scott Base.'

'Yeah Scott Base, K001-Bravo, checking in for our evening sked, we have nine people out here and everything is perfect, over.'

I'm sitting on the other side of the entrance from Richard. Our tent, it is pointed out to me, is a bit of luxury—we're 'glamping in the Friis Hills,' someone says. In one corner of the tent a diesel-fuelled heater keeps the air above freezing point. On top of the heater a large pot melts snow and heats the water to boiling for tea, soup, instant noodles, and Cliff's hot Raro. At the same end of the tent are two Coleman stoves, each with two gas burners, and a collection of pots, pans and cooking equipment.

In the middle of the tent is the large trestle table, covered in cups and thermos flasks, maps and cameras, sunblock, and snacks—biscuits, crackers, peanuts and muesli bars. We sit on folding chairs around the edge of the tent, crowded amid boxes of gear that needs to be protected from the outside cold—the radio equipment, computers, electronic field gear, the food we don't want frozen. It's a tight fit, and there are a lot of excuse me's as people move from one end of the tent to the other to get a hot drink, retrieve a notebook or pop outside to the loo.

But even here in the Polar Haven, heated by the stove

to a steady 7°C or so and with everything *perfect*, I'm still uncomfortable and on edge. I can feel the cold seeping up from the ground and into my legs. I'm used to being a highly competent human. Here I feel almost useless. I'm breathing badly. I'm cold. I'm slow. All day people have been offering to help me with things, carry something, offer me a hand, and I'm not used to it.

We had a few days of sunny, settled weather down at Scott Base. But here at our camp, in the mountains, it's getting colder and the barometric pressure is dropping. Outside, the wind is blowing and the snow is getting heavier.

'Friis Hills is about to bare its ugly teeth,' says Warren.

'979 we're down to, now. It's dropping through the floor,' says Nick, looking at the barometer on his watch.

This tiny campsite has become my world. I love snow, but the fact that we are now cut off from Scott Base and McMurdo Station—what stands for civilisation around here—gives me a surge of claustrophobia. We really are stuck here.

Dinner is 'Mexican pile', made by Adam. A crumble of corn chips topped with a chilli meat and bean mixture and cheese. A kind of hearty nachos, heavy on the chilli. We follow dinner with some Glenlivet whisky served with ice chips cut from a chunk of the ice Cliff brought up from the Taylor Glacier. There are satellite photographs of Friis Hills on the table and everyone is talking about fieldwork logistics—the challenges of drilling in the permafrost and running seismic lines in the snow.

Every now and then there's a break in the chatter and it's quiet except for the gentle roar of the stove and the occasional flap of the tent in the wind. Everyone's a bit slow because of the cold. Sitting still, heads bent, eyes down. Then someone pipes up with the often repeated, usually ironic, 'She's a harsh continent', and conversation resumes.

'Happy to be here, lucky to be here,' someone says.

The guys are still planning the next day's fieldwork, but I need to be on my own so I say my goodnights and head for my tent through the bright white of the blowing snow.

The surface beneath the snow is dusty and brown and every time I go into my tent I track in a bit of 14-million-year-old dirt mixed with fresh snow. Getting in and out of the tent, which has a flysheet over the top, is a mission. Because of the cold, I'm wearing my Extreme Cold Weather boots and I need to take them off before crawling inside. It's a one-person tent, and inside is my three-layer sleeping bag—a down bag inside a synthetic bag inside a canvas bag—on top of my foam and sheepskin sleeping mats. Beside the bed, my clothes and books are spilling out of a large stuff bag. My pee bottle is in one corner of the tent and my drink bottle is in another (note to self: do not mix them up). I'm a messy traveller, and my tendency to fling things from one end of the tent to another is not good here, as the mixture of dust from outside and moisture from melting snow is making things mucky. I wasn't expecting dirt in Antarctica.

I strip off everything except my thermals, socks, hat and neck gaiter and get as deep into my bags as I can. Despite the time—it's after nine o'clock—and the falling snow, it's light. The sun won't set here for another three months and there's a gentle orange glow inside my tent. It's cosy, and I usually cherish alone time, but I'm having trouble breathing and I'm starting to panic.

On my own in the tent, without any chatter around me, I acknowledge to myself that I really don't feel good. My head is buzzing. My chest feels tight and my heart is palpitating. I can't breathe.

I don't know if there is something physically wrong with me or if it's anxiety. My father is dying. My fixed-term contract at the university is about to come to an end. I've been on the go—all work, no play—for two years solid and I think my body has forgotten how to relax. To make it worse, my kids didn't want me to leave home. I've been away a lot during the last two years—to academic conferences, and back and forth to see my father in the United States where he was having treatment, and once he moved back to New Zealand, to Christchurch—and at some level I feel selfish and bad for being away again.

What the fuck am I doing here?

I take stock. I'm alone in a small tent on an ice-free plateau in the Dry Valleys region of Antarctica. It's −20°C and there's a light snow falling, making a gentle pittering sound, like someone is throwing small handfuls of sand at my tent. Nearby in the Polar Haven tent, the geologists are gathered around the stove, chatting and having one last drink before bedtime.

The geologists are my friends—I trust them and like them—but I'm too ashamed to reveal how on edge I feel. I'm so privileged to be here. But I'm feeling trapped. There's no warm 'inside' I can escape to. If I'm sick, there's no chance of a medevac as the helicopters can't fly in a blizzard.

Some people do lose it up here in the Dry Valleys; it's the cold climate version of going troppo. The other night Tim told a story about a team camped in a nearby valley radioing in with a 'send more Valium' request. Instead of sending more Valium, they sent a helicopter to remove the afflicted young scientist. I have a small vial of Diazepam, a benzodiazepine similar to Valium, but in this unfamiliar situation I'm too anxious to take it. If my symptoms are not anxiety, if they're something else, I worry that taking Diazepam in this cold, at this altitude, might have unintended consequences. It might be contraindicated, so I continue without it, in case it masks physical symptoms that will be needed to diagnose me. I'm aware that I'm being overdramatic but it doesn't help how I feel.

I try some mindfulness techniques. I focus on the orange of the tent, the sound of the dry snow hitting the nylon, the feeling of the cold air on my face, and I become aware of my tiredness.

At home I sometimes lie awake at night and worry—panic, even—about climate change and what we're doing to the planet and the future world my children will grow up in. Tonight I try to focus on my breathing, using a technique taught to me by a respiratory physiotherapist. I try to think about how I'm going to get warm, whether my water is going to stay unfrozen, and whether I need to use my pee bottle before I go to sleep.

There's nothing more I can do. If I die tonight, then I die tonight. I think about the absurdity of this thought and the unlikeliness of it and I sleep.

The next day I let on to Tim that I've been feeling 'a bit breathless'. 'It could just be the excitement . . .' I suggest, and trail off, avoiding the word 'anxiety'. These guys are so great for inviting me. I don't want to be negative.

Tim is attentive but unfazed and suggests it's 'cold asthma'. 'I get it sometimes,' he adds. The shock of the cold, dry air, combined with high altitude, can irritate the lungs and constrict the breathing passages, causing a form of asthma that can hit people who otherwise do not suffer from the condition. It's not that high here—1300 metres at our camp, 1700 metres at the highest point of the hills—but at this high latitude (77.45°S) the air pressure is even lower. I feel grateful to have a possible physical explanation for my breathlessness and reassured to know there is treatment if I need it. Tim has an asthma inhaler in the medicine chest, along with Valium, morphine, antibiotics and more. I'm relieved. I feel I can get on with my day now, but it does get me thinking about my father. I hope the doctors have fixed his medication so that he's free of pain and clearer in his head.

It's stopped snowing now, so while four of the geologists are setting up the seismic line, Adam takes the rest of us—Warren, Cliff, Christoph and me—for a walk. I ditch my ECW boots for Sorels, which are much more comfortable for walking.

Although the snow has disguised the landscape he's so familiar with, Adam can see paths he's made on previous visits and we walk east towards a spot where Cliff wants to look at an outcrop of basement rock. As we walk, Adam tells us about the geology, and his past trips here, and I'm happily distracted from my symptoms, whether they're physical or psychosomatic.

Adam and his students have identified a sequence of Friis Hills glacial moraines interspersed with life-supporting water bodies—ponds, marshes and small lakes—created by glacial meltwaters. About 14 million years ago the climate changed: air temperatures became colder, rain stopped falling and the water became locked up in glacial ice—plants could no longer grow here. At least that's what the geomorphologists believe.

From a high point—one of the hills that give Friis Hills its name—we have a view across the Taylor Glacier to the steep-sided Kukri Hills, a 2000-metre-high range that separates the Taylor from the Ferrar Glacier. Beyond the western edge of the hills, we can see across some 20 kilometres of ice that feeds both the Taylor and Ferrar Glaciers. Beyond that, are the 4000-metre-high peaks of the Royal Society Range. The sun is shining, the visibility seemingly endless. The view of the layered brown cliffs, distant mountain peaks, and the flat white glacier is . . . stupendous, jaw-dropping, awe-inspiring, cliché-inducing. Later that day I review some video footage of Cliff talking in front of the mountains and glaciers, and the light in the footage is so perfect and the sound of his voice so clear that it seems fake, as if recorded in front of a studio green screen.

As we continue our walk, Adam stops and points to some parallel indents on the ground, more than a metre apart, in-filled by the new snow. I wonder if they're a geological feature, but Adam says they're marks left by a very heavy helicopter, the type of old military machine that used to fly around here in the decades after International Geophysical Year, which spanned the summer of 1957 and 1958 and saw bases built—

including Scott Base and McMurdo Station—and an expansion of Antarctic science and exploration. You often find old smoke canisters around here too, says Adam, used to indicate wind direction to helicopter pilots. Today, everything that goes into the field comes out of the field—there'd be no chance of crew throwing their stuff on the ground and leaving it—but there is still some rubbish and detritus left over from earlier days before the Antarctic Environmental Protocol was signed in 1991.

Around the corner is what Cliff has come to see, an unconformity where a yellow-brown conglomerate, deposited 420 million years ago by an ancient river system, sits directly on top of a 500-million-year-old granite. The conglomerate is part of the Beacon Supergroup, a thick layer of sediment that includes coals, fish fossils and tree fragments. Cliff films a clip—he talks about deep time, geological evidence, reading the rocks—then we stop for lunch. There's a pile of dolerite boulders and we use them variously as seats, leaning posts, tables. I've brought a packet of crackers and a can of tuna, more than I want so I offer them around. I drink from my water bottle. I'm drinking a lot, but am relieved that I don't need to pee yet. Not quite as easy for me as it is for the others.

As we walk back, the guys are discussing past experiences of Antarctic fieldwork. There are stories of frostnip, epic storms, gung-ho helicopter pilots flying in white-outs. But it's a gorgeous day here now, the sun is shining and there is barely a breeze.

Walking the landscape, just looking and thinking, is a big part of what Adam does as a geomorphologist. 'It takes me a week or two to actually start to see everything,' he says. 'The first two weeks, I'm blind, then all of a sudden I see things I'd walked right through before. It's like all your distractions and thinking about other things disappears, and you start to really notice details and patterns, and sort of read the landscape.'

What sort of details, I ask?

'Say you're walking along on a rocky, armoured surface and there are six rock types that make it up. Well, you walk a little bit and all of a sudden there aren't six rock types, there are five. Normally you would never notice that but if you're out there all the time and all you're doing is looking at the ground as you walk, then looking up at the hills, then back at the ground, you're going to notice and go "hey, that rock is missing". Now that would not happen the first week, it probably wouldn't happen the first couple of weeks. It takes a while to sort of forget the other distractions.' Details like this can signify the end of one glacial deposit and the start of another.

This year the snow is obscuring the sorts of clues that Adam would normally see, but he's still attentive and I envy him this focus on the landscape, on the here and now, his ability to be where he is. All the geologists seem to have this. They are intimately connected to the environment around them, the instruments they're using, rather than being caught up in their own heads like I usually am. Maybe it's my constant need to translate what I'm experiencing into words, to find or create a narrative, that stops me fully engaging with my surroundings. I'm constantly jumping from the world around me to my inner world, always aware that I might try and write my experience into something that non-scientists can read.

On our walk, Adam apologises to me when he swears. And when he clears his nose by holding one nostril and blowing out the other he says he hopes I don't find it too disgusting here. But . . . it's beautiful here! I think to myself. I blow my nose like that too, on occasion, if necessary, and for want of better adjectives my inner monologue and my journals are incredibly sweary. I am surprised at the degree to which he's misinterpreted me, or that I'm misrepresenting myself. I've withdrawn into myself in the cold and become someone else.

—

While we've been walking, the rest of the team have been setting up a seismic line. The aim is to use this remote geophysical method to find the depth of the basement rocks that lie beneath the lake and glacial sediments. Results from the seismic line will be used to determine the best places to drill to get cores that contain many millions of years of deposits. The aim is to get a seismic line extending the full 5 kilometres across the Friis Hills basin.

As we get close to camp we can see Andrew the geophysicist huddling over his computer screen, sitting on the upturned equipment box. He has his ECW jacket draped over him and his computer, trying to darken the screen so he can see it in the bright sunlight.

Andrew usually has a couple of second-year undergraduates doing his seismic lines but this time he has Tim, Richard, Nick and Christoph. They've laid out a set of black and yellow cables extending from his seismometer across the valley floor, with a geophone placed every five metres. When a noise is made on the surface, some of the sound waves travel through the sediments and bounce back off any harder layer underneath. The geophones pick up the returning sound waves and relay the signal back to the seismometer and into Andrew's laptop. While some seismic surveys use explosions to create the sound, this is a 'hammer seismic' survey and makes use of a sledgehammer, a metal plate, and some muscle.

We walk down the line to where Richard and Nick are waiting for Andrew to tell them to start. Once we're close we need to stand still, so we don't add any noise to the signal.

'Quiet on the line,' we hear Andrew's voice through one of the VHF radios we use to communicate across short distances—anywhere you can get a direct line from one radio to the next.

'On station,' Richard replies.

'Fire when ready,' says Andrew.

Nick swings the sledgehammer onto a metal plate five

times—*tink!*—while Richard counts 'one-one-thousand, two-one-thousand' to time each swing.

Andrew has been watching the trace on his computer screen. 'That looks good,' we hear him say. 'Move to next station'.

It's heavy work swinging the hammer and Nick and Richard—both of them strong and lean and over six foot tall—take turns with it. For Andrew, it's monotonous work, sitting, watching, and issuing instructions by radio.

'Whack away,' he continues.

Tim and Christoph—who, because of his toilet duties, is now generally referred to as 'Scheisse Boy'—are laying out the next section of seismic line. I keep offering to help. I should at least be able to carry something from one place to another. I can't really be any worse than a geology student, but I am. I feel kind of useless, I hope I'm not getting in people's way. I'm actually starting to feel sorry for myself.

'I think this will be a juicy little drilling target, this basin,' says Tim, after assuring me they don't need my help.

It's too cold for me. I feel miserable. Cliff and I do some more filming and I get even colder just standing behind the camera. Eventually Cliff notices that I'm not okay and sends me back to the Polar Haven to warm up. Once he's finished his to-camera he joins me. The problem, he thinks, is that I'm not eating enough to keep warm. It turns out my plan to starve out my imagined tummy bug was deranged. My tummy wasn't upset; I was just nervous. Cliff passes me a cup of hot Raro and a handful of biscuits and tells me to get it down me. Some frozen lollies, and some cheese and salami later—fats and sugars—and I start feeling a bit better.

While dinner is cooking I finally work up the courage—necessity is a key part of it—to go to the open-air loo. I trudge past a yellow tent and down the path made by all our footsteps. The side of the loo facing the tents is a stack of dolerite slabs, about chest high—if someone is sitting down, all you can see is the top of their head. The loo itself is a yellow plastic bucket filled with a large plastic bag and topped with a foam seat and a bucket lid. On top of the lid is a slab of rock, to ensure that nothing blows away. Next to the loo, a roll of paper and a bottle of hand sanitiser are wedged between two rocks. Next to all this are the white plastic pee barrels. Lots of them. The one in active use has a funnel on top. For the guys, it's a simple matter of aiming into the funnel. If I was game at using the Shee-wee—the 'female urination device' I was issued with in Christchurch—I could stand and attempt the same, but I prefer to use a pee bottle in the privacy of my tent and come tip it in here when it's full.

Anyway, I raise the black flag on a bamboo pole to indicate the loo is in use, take the rock off the seat, and pull down my over-trousers and thermals. I'm sitting there, pants down, looking at a pretty spectacular view but hoping that this will all be over quickly—it's −20°C for fuck's sake, and it feels very weird to be so exposed—when I hear footsteps and Tim's voice. 'Oh shit, sorry!'

He sounds mortified.

'Didn't you see the black flag?!' I yell back at him. We had a system!

He walks back to camp. I hear him bust into the Polar Haven with a 'Jesus fuckin' Christ, I just walked in on Rebecca.'

When I get back to the tent, I've got to a place somewhere beyond embarrassment, a place where I have no ego. There are no barriers. One of the worst things that I could imagine has happened, and I feel relaxed. Whatever.

'Tim fuckin' Naish,' I say as I enter the Polar Haven, newly confident now that I've dealt to my hunger. It goes without saying that I own him now, and he shuffles around the table and hands me a beer.

But people won't let it alone, and soon the main topic of

conversation is Antarctic toilet experiences. There's a story about a piece of wind-blown, poo-streaked toilet paper that a field trainer had to retrieve from high up a cliff. Another about Lake Chad, a small lake further down the Taylor Valley. People tend to think it was named after the country or a person, but it turns out it was named for a brand of toilet paper, after a team led by Australian geologist Griffith Taylor camped there in 1911 and all got the runs. Or so I'm told.

Tim and I are now the butt of a series of jokes. I don't mind. These guys are fun and funny and I'm happy. I've spent the day walking in an Antarctic snowscape, in full sunshine, and talking about geology. There have been no emergency calls—my children seem to be surviving without me and my father hasn't died. Perhaps I could relax just a little bit, let go and try to enjoy things while I am relatively free from my usual responsibilities.

I help make dinner of stir-fried chicken and vegetables with rice. Warren makes margaritas—Jose Cuervo Especial, Triple Sec and Rose's lime juice—in an aluminium cooking pot.

'There's a bit of Antarctic experience in this tent,' says Richard as we eat. We count it up. Between the nine of us, are eight PhDs and 60 Antarctic seasons.

After dinner Cliff holds up a hinged wooden box—the words 'Macinlay's Rare Old Highland Malt Whisky' is painted on the side and 'British Antarctic Expedition 1907' on one end—and asks everyone to pay attention. 'If you don't know the story,' he says, 'they found some whisky under Shackleton's hut a few years ago and a few of the bottles were still in good condition. So they took them back to New Zealand, then they got a distillery in Scotland to recreate the whisky.' Inside the box, the bottle rests on a bed of straw. 'Apparently it's not that great a whisky,' he says, 'but the story is good.' This is Cliff's second $200 bottle of Shackleton whisky. The first one, he tells us, he drank up on the Nansen Ice Shelf the previous season. Tim tried some a few weeks earlier with a colleague in Illinois.

I first tried the whisky, with my sister Rachel, at an Antarctic Heritage Trust tasting in Wellington back in 2011. We bought a bottle for Dad, but I think it's still sitting in his cabinet.

Cliff unwraps the bottle, strips off the foil and pulls out the cork—plip! 'Who'd like some?' People drain the last of their margaritas then pass forward their cups—a brightly coloured jumble of plastic insulated mugs.

'No sipping until we have the toast,' says Tim. 'Just hold on to it.'

The next few minutes are caught up in arguments over the best way to break cup-friendly pieces of ice off our diminishing chunk of Taylor Glacier ice —we have 'a bit of an ice issue,' says someone—but soon there's a piece for everyone. We all lumber—in our heavy coats and over-trousers there's no chance of swift movement—to our feet.

Cliff raises his cup and thanks the geology team for inviting us along. 'Pleased to be here, lucky to be here, happy to be here, so yeah, cheers to that,' he says.

Then Nick proposes a toast to the 'old explorers'. Christoph says a big thank you for being taken on his first trip to Antarctica, and Cliff toasts his dad, whose birthday is the next day. There's a big round of 'Cheers' and clumsy clunks as we try to touch plastic cups across the table.

It's not as nice as the Glenlivet we were drinking the night before.

'It's pretty cool though,' says Richard, 'that we're drinking the same thing that old Shackleton drank.'

'I know! And out of the same mugs,' adds someone.

The foolish banter continues—theories about the left-behind bottles of whisky morph into tales of Scott Base antics from previous Antarctic seasons—and with the mixture of relief at no longer feeling so cold, my newfound loss of ego, and the drinks I find myself laughing until I cry. I cover my face, wipe away tears, but the jokes and stories continue and my laughter keeps coming. I feel like a second-year student on a geology field trip.

We're all tired. Adam sings a few lines from a Johnny Cash song—*I hear the train a comin' rollin' round the bend / I ain't seen the sunshine since I don't know when*—then, after some silence, Richard starts quietly singing Rolf Harris's 'Two Little Boys'—a song I haven't heard since I was a kid—and Tim joins in. Everyone has a mug in their hands. Heads bowed, gazing down into nothing. I slip out of the Polar Haven while I'm still feeling good and crawl into my little orange tent.

The sun is shining. I'm settled into my sleeping bag. I can hear the guys talking; they're up on the ridge now, drinking whisky, looking at the mountains across the glacier. I'm kind of wishing I was up there with them but it was time for me to go to bed. The tension between not wanting to miss out on anything and knowing that I need time alone, time downloading my thoughts and impressions and feelings, is always there, on every trip I'm on.

I'm happy and sad at the same time. As soon as I've warmed up and started to feel comfortable here, I'm going to have to leave. As I listen to the chatter from the ridge above me, I think about how these scientists—whether they're operating geophysical equipment, walking and interpreting the landscape, or just drinking whisky and looking at the view—seem good at living in the moment. At the same time, though, they're dealing with deep geological time and working on problems with implications for the future of humanity. I wonder if their work gives them a sense of perspective that makes day-to-day living easier.

I wake the next morning happy and warm. I have no idea what time it is. The sun has been shining all night and my iPhone—my only means of telling the time—gave up in the cold. It went from 100 percent power to shutting off. I'm beginning to like it here.

The air inside the tent feels mild, but it's deceptive—the water in my drink bottle is frozen, so 'warm' has become a relative thing. Planning is important here. It's crucial to hold on to the warmth that you start the day with. If you go outside and get cold it's very hard to get back that heat. I don't think about how I feel—warm—but what I know—my water bottle is frozen—and I plan to conserve every bit of heat. So before I climb out of my sleeping bag I put on a woollen jersey and fleece jacket over my thermal top. I jump out of my bag and pull up my socks so there's no skin gap between socks and thermals. I pee in the bottle then put on another jacket, my over-trousers and my boots and head for the Polar Haven.

Soon after breakfast some TV people arrive by helicopter wearing goggles and neck gaiters and with their fur-lined hoods pulled tight. Perhaps I have acclimatised. There are three of them, all lively and important. A producer, a camera operator, and a glamorous presenter whom I escort to my little orange tent—she'll be sleeping here for the next few nights. She's slimmer than me and vegetarian, and I wonder how she'll cope in the cold. I find myself slightly envious that I'm leaving and she's staying. Cliff and I help carry their stuff—there's lot of it, their camera gear is much bigger than ours—from the landing spot to the campsite. Richard, Nick and Andrew are off doing their seismic line.

The helicopter is our ride back to Scott Base, but not just yet. Warren and Cliff climb on board and head back to Marble Point to refuel then Sean flies the chopper low to the ground, back and forth over the Friis Hills in a planned grid transect. Warren hangs out of the open door, his feet on the skids and body as far forward as he can while still sitting on the seat, taking photographs of the ground. He is wearing a harness, which is clipped into the back of the chopper, but Cliff's providing back up, a pair of strong hands holding onto Warren's harness as an extra point of safety.

Tim is playing host, showing the TV people around the camp and making them a cuppa. While we're all sitting inside the Polar Haven, there's a call on the VHF radio—Nick, who's on the seismic line, needs the GPS receiver to plot their location. The one Tim has in his pocket. I offer to run it down to the line. It's close in the tent and despite my newly attained sense of wellbeing it is a fragile wellness and I don't feel like being around bubbly TV people and Antarctic newbies.

I deliver the GPS to Nick and head towards camp along a trail of footsteps in the snow. I don't want to go back to camp just now so I stop, sit on a lump of dolerite deposited there by a glacier millions of years ago, and cry. I feel as if I've barely engaged with the fact that I'm here, camping in the mountains of Antarctica. I'm so happy to be here—lucky to be here—but when I get home my father will still be dying, I'll have to re-apply for the job I've been doing for two years, I'll have to compensate at home for being away for two weeks, and I won't have time to sit on a rock and look at the world around me. It feels right to be crying. It feels like the only way I can respond to this landscape and how I'm feeling inside and what I'm heading home to.

I take a deep breath and manage, for the first time on this trip, to be fully here, alone. I'm looking out on a landscape that could almost be Mars. A landscape that tells a story of a warmer Antarctica, with lakes and rivers, and insects buzzing around the trees. Sun glistens on the snow. On the ground, coloured pebbles and rocks rise above the white surface. There used to be a thick layer of glacial moraine here, a pile of sand and dust and rocks and boulders more than 30 metres deep, but wind has blown almost all of it away. This is a deflation landscape, a landscape of loss.

There's a distant crack of the sledgehammer on the metal plate. Then I hear the chopper coming back. It's time to leave.

Water Wings

Sarah Lin Wilson

When I was seven, my hair started falling out. My father would brush it, and I'd watch as thin strands drifted to the floor. When it was wet, it formed a straight helmet around my head, and my brothers teased me for looking like Darth Vader. That was the first time I can remember crying because I felt I wasn't 'normal'.

I read a lot as a kid, and anxiety was one of those words I learned the look of before I learned its sound. I knew how to say 'anxious', though not what it meant—so I extrapolated from that and came up with 'anxious-tee'. It didn't occur to me that I might be experiencing anxious-tee. I knew I worried. I knew I was afraid of things that other people weren't. I knew I was somehow *different*, but I had no word or reason for that difference.

The worrying got worse as I grew, and most of the time it had little logical basis. I felt sick a lot. I found myself panicking when the sun went down, because night-time frightened me—the time, not the darkness. I developed compulsive behaviours to try to control the world: counting things in even numbers, needing layers of heavy blankets on my bed in a certain order, wanting the same foods every day. It felt like if I didn't stick to these routines, the world would implode.

One day after intermediate school, I got in the car with my father and told him I felt sick.

'I feel like I'm nervous, Dad,' I said. It was the sort of nervous you get before doing a speech in English class when you're a painfully shy child who prefers writing poems in the library than talking to people. But I didn't have any speeches to do—there was nothing obvious to be nervous about. My father, himself an anxious person and soon to be a qualified counsellor, told me what I felt was called anxiety, and it was okay to feel this way, even though it wasn't fun. There were ways to manage it, he said. So began my journey to find them.

I was lucky enough to have an understanding and supportive family. I was always encouraged to talk about my feelings at home. This didn't stop me from worrying, but I quickly learned that putting how I felt into words could help create fences around feelings that seemed huge and boundless. The same was true for writing, which provided relief and solace.

When I left Nelson to go to university in Wellington, contact with my family became difficult—everyone was still on dial-up internet, and calling from my cellphone cost about as much as a week's worth of groceries. I battled the increased anxieties of academic pressure, socialising and learning how to be an independent adult, along with what I now know to be depression.

After a year of worsening panic and mood swings, I was finally persuaded to try medication. I'd battled internally with the stigma around needing it; I had to fight the belief that it somehow made me weak. In hindsight, it took courage to make the choice. I trialled a few antidepressants before I found one that seemed to help. Nothing stopped the anxiety or magically made me happy, but now I was able to control my symptoms. I started working at the National Library while I finished my communications degree.

I found the best way of quelling anxiety was to excel at work. Academic and professional achievement gave me an endorphin rush. I felt valid and valued. I was a workaholic, and I was happy.

In 2012, I decided to move back to Nelson to spend time with my family and work freelance. What I hadn't foreseen was that, when you're self-employed and anxious, you work 24/7.

I couldn't stop: I was always 'on', and so was my anxiety. I developed bad habits, like working through dinner, working till midnight, working in the weekends. I was trying to outrun the anxiety. Unfortunately for me, anxiety never sleeps.

I'm often reminded of that movie *Rat Race*, where Rowan Atkinson plays a narcoleptic. 'It's a race it's a race it's a race,' he hollers, running with his arms in the air—then passes out and falls over on the spot.

In March 2013, I collapsed and was hospitalised. Unbeknownst to me, my body had been fighting an infection called *Clostridium difficile*, caused by me taking too many antibiotics so that I could continue working. *C. diff* is nasty. But even when throwing up in a bucket beside my bed, I had my laptop on my knee. I answered my phone from hospital and pretended to be in the office. My anxiety would not let me let go.

In the months following hospitalisation, my mood disorders were close to the worst they've ever been. I was extremely fatigued—most days, I could move from the bed to the couch and back, and that would be all. After months of waiting for the recovery that my doctors told me would come, I finally admitted I needed to stop working. Conversations exhausted me. *Thinking* exhausted me. I had more than burned out. There was nothing left of me but a vague impression in soot.

And because I could not *achieve* in the way I was used to, I could not control the upwards spiralling of my anxiety or the downwards spiralling of my mood. I tried to be patient, but pain became more and more of my daily routine. This was new pain, in my joints and pelvis and spine. I queried the doctors and was given the same edict again: patience.

More than a year later I was diagnosed with inflammatory autoimmune arthritis—Ankylosing Spondylitis (AS)—a genetic condition which had been triggered by the inflammation of the *C. diff*. Having AS means that my immune system attacks parts of my body that are actually healthy, leaving me in widespread pain and fatigue. Some days, I can go a couple of hours without thinking about how much I hurt or how much I want to go back to bed. Others, I feel like I am 90 years old. I am 31.

'Comorbidity' means that certain illnesses are likely to go hand in hand. I have yet to find anyone with a chronic illness or disability like mine who does not also suffer from mental illness. Unfortunately, this makes sense.

Having experienced anxiety and depression for a long time, I had methods of dealing with them that weren't perfect, but they helped. AS dramatically altered my ability to do them; I had to reduce the freelance work that fed my self-esteem, the socialising that built my morale, the exercise that helped burn nervous energy and replace it with endorphins.

My physical circumstances also fed my anxiety that I would absolutely and continuously let people down. I lay in bed running lists through my head, torturing myself with the fact that I couldn't cross anything off. I couldn't *achieve* things, and therefore I could never calm my anxiety or boost my self-esteem to fight off depression. My perfectionism became my worst enemy.

Slowly, I regained some strength and was able to resume basic activities. But it became clear that I wasn't going to be working full-time any time soon. I needed to find another way of coping with my need to achieve.

In 1962, Australian doctor and researcher Dr Claire Weekes wrote the book *Self Help for Your Nerves*, in which she talks about how to recover from a nervous breakdown. There's a picture of Dr Weekes on the inside of the cover. She looks like someone's grandmother, and her advice is fittingly gentle and no-nonsense.

I wasn't recovering from a breakdown, not in the sense she talks of, but some of her advice stands, despite being over 50 years old. My 'nerves' were the challenge; after all these years, I was still the 12-year-old with butterflies.

Dr Weekes's solution is simple, on the surface. She calls it 'floating'. In today's psychological lexicon, that's mindfulness and acceptance. She encourages patients to float towards or past their difficulties. The key to recovery, she says, is to stop fighting.

Predictably, I fought this idea. I was furious. I buried the book at the bottom of my to-read pile. I'd spent my whole life fighting: to suppress my anxiety, to live a 'normal' life in *spite* of it, to pretend it didn't exist. To *stop* fighting felt like giving in, and there was no way I wanted the anxiety to win. But I wasn't winning, either. Not only was my fighting not working—it was making me more ill. I didn't have the physical or mental energy to keep it up. Something had to give.

Acceptance should feel calm. But, for me, getting there involved a freefall of terror first, like trying to float past a rip in the tide. How was I supposed to accept this anxiety when I felt that I needed to escape the swirling vortex so I wouldn't be sucked under? Mindfulness has never worked for me, though I've tried meditation courses and apps. The concept is appealing, but paying attention to the present moment doesn't calm me. Instead, I've learned my own way of floating, which involves something like doggy paddle and water wings.

Recognising my reduced capacity was the first step. I haven't lowered my expectations for how well I will do something—I've just capped the number of things I do. Instead of trying for 20 laps of the pool, I do two—and then go sit in the spa. I still get a feeling of achievement, even though I've had to reduce my list of accomplishments. Acceptance means being kind to yourself.

Acceptance also involves not turning down assistance. Sometimes it's easier to stay afloat when someone offers an arm. It took me a while to learn that taking their hand isn't giving in; it's fighting in a different way. If the only way I can get through is by letting someone drive me to an appointment or cook a meal, refusing those things isn't strong. It's stubborn, and it's a guaranteed way of going under. In a shocking turn of events (ha), I realised that my friends actually wanted to be my friends. They accepted me, and I learned to accept them.

It's hard to know if I'm floating in the way that Dr Weekes really meant—I think one of her examples involved drifting past a bakery, and I've never done that in my life. In any case, I'm not stuck in the vortex, and I'm not standing still. So, even if my trip to the pool mainly means a trip to the spa, I'm okay with that. I haven't stopped fighting the anxious-tee, not completely. But I've accepted that, for me, boxing gloves look a lot more like water wings.

What Happens

Zion Tauamiti

I didn't ever dream of being this guy. I never studied to be a suicide prevention officer; I never wanted to be one when I was a kid. I was led to the job. This is my vocation. It's hard to say how I got into it. I'm a really spiritual guy, and I love working with people and finding solutions. Why do it? Because I'm sensitive to how I think the wairua, the spirit, is leading me. Because I'm hungry to see change. But when you're working on a scale where, at one end, someone might die, how do you create this change? What are the solutions, answers, alternatives to suicide? My job is basically to find out what will help the kids want to stay alive.

I developed a mental health and wellbeing programme. It was like a fruit salad: you'd say, I'll take all of them, I'll take anyone who's struggling with whatever. Our main aim was suicide prevention, and I spent a lot of time talking kids through their anxiety. Whenever someone was having a panic attack, their anxiety triggered to the next level, I would guide them through it; say, Okay, do this. Breathe. Panic attacks are like anxiety on steroids. Sometimes the kid would be hyperventilating, or they'd start screaming, really hysterical.

It was horrible. Oh my gosh, it was horrible watching them. Anxiety is really easy to identify. The certain tics, behaviours. It's so different from depression; it's its own thing. Some of the kids would talk heaps, just non-stop verbal diarrhoea—a coping mechanism when they're scared. If I was sitting with somebody who was continuously talking, I'd be like, straight out, Hey, how is your anxiety? Or if I was in a car with a kid who was constantly looking around, checking their surroundings, hyper-alert. I'd ask, Are you okay? And they'd tell me what was happening to them. I'd have to reassure them that they were okay, that they were safe.

I worked with all kids. I played a role where I was like a visitor, an uncle. Parents do their best, but they aren't always in a position to help. Often family members and friends around the kid get over it. They think, Oh, I just can't be bothered dealing with them. I've seen people give up on them, say Yeah, nah. This just perpetuates the anxiety, because for the kid it's like, Oh, there's no point in asking for help. No point in telling people. Every time I tell someone I'm struggling, I get shut down. So I'm not going to tell anyone.

Sometimes you'd get to see the best sides of these kids, and sometimes you'd see the ugliest. I try to look back at when I was a teenager—which was ages ago, 15 years—and I remember those days were horrible. Always worrying about the peer pressure, trying to keep up the facade. I can see why the kids lose their rag all the time or are full of anxiety. Especially today. Social media contributes heaps to kids' sense of worth and self. I think that's massive. The hits to their self-esteem are everywhere, particularly for young women. They're the filter generation, and they are constantly questioning their images, their value to the world beyond that. Boys have their own struggles. Especially young athletes. They always have to be really masculine, all good, staunch. Lying.

Sexual pressure is huge. It's one of the biggest contributing factors to suicide. Anxiety can be one of the interim stops along the way to that decision. It's emotional purgatory. Some people have had a traumatic experience during childhood, and that's life-altering. Especially when it's anything sexual. That damages your brain. You're always worried about who's around you, or nervous about the dark. You can't sleep. For heaps of our girls, the triggers are the same: if you go to sleep, you might wake up to find someone on top of you. Can you imagine?

Sleeping being a dangerous place?

This one case in particular. A year 10 girl whose friend brought her to me and said, She's suicidal, she's been talking about it heaps. That's when the real work starts, when you have to sit with someone. If they're sitting with you, you should feel honoured, eh. You're already halfway to meeting their needs. They're talking you through their story and you have to be super alert and pick up on things. You look at them and you say, What's happening? And they say, I've got anxiety.

When do you reckon that started?

When I was 12 I started, like, feeling suicidal and I was anxious every day.

Oh yep. So you said it started when you were 12. What happened when you were 12?

Oh, well, you know, my sister's partner abused me. It started there.

Oh. Okay. Did you tell the police?

Yes, I told the police.

Did you go to court?

Yes, I went to court.

What happened in court?

They dismissed it and threw it out. Said there wasn't enough evidence.

How did it make you feel?

It made me feel like I don't have a voice. Like why am I even fucking here? Why am I alive? I should just be dead.

Another girl was a singer and she ended up on the youth mental health ward. I went to visit her. She had a speech impediment, something was wrong with her voice. I said, What happened? She couldn't speak properly, but she was trying to explain it to me. She told me that she was raped in the school holidays, and then one day she was at school and they were talking about rape in assembly, which triggered the fuck out of her, and she started having a seizure. They had to ring the ambulance and it came to get her, and one of the side effects of the seizure was this speech thing. I was like, Okay, I'm sorry about that. So can you still sing? She said, I don't know. I played a song she loved and she started singing, and she could pronounce all the words. Her diction was great. I'm like, what the hell, you can't talk but you can sing? That's anxiety.

I met someone who couldn't sleep with the light off. Couldn't sleep in the dark. She was 16 years old, and she said, I don't feel safe. I always have to have the lamp on. So I asked, What happened?

Something happened in the dark.

What happened in the dark?

I was this old. My dad is an alcoholic and all his mates were around and one of his mates walked through the door and says, Sorry, I thought this was the toilet. But closes the door. Locks the door.

That's anxiety. It's like waiting to get a hiding. Me as a kid, my anxiety was around if I was naughty and I knew I was going to get a hiding. And it's so crippling. Waiting to be abused, for that event that changed your life to happen again. That's all you know: waiting to be told you're shit, waiting to fail. So you walk about with this stuff crushing your skull. You go home and it's stressful at home and you're not heard there. You go to school and it's all crazy and you're not heard there.

So, okay, these kids feel anxious because they feel unsafe because they feel they don't belong, because they're unheard. They just need a voice. They need to be heard. So let's set up environments and safe places, create spaces where kids can actually be heard. I think you can do that anywhere, but it depends on the experience that originally made them feel unsafe. If their family life is unsafe, or if it's their father or mother, you pick up on that real quick and you say, Okay, you have a dad who yells at you, he's never proud of you and tells you you're shit. Okay, cool. I'm proud of you. It's getting in their head and giving their brain a cuddle, telling them they're okay. It's hard watching it. It's really sad.

Schools are calling out for people who can help. Teachers referred kids to me. Teachers have heaps of shit on their plates as it is, and in those frontline jobs nowadays you're not just a teacher or a policeman—you actually need to be a social worker as well. It's stressful for them. I get teachers talking to me all the time saying, I didn't ask for this. It's hard for the ones who are the first port of call, the firefighters, teachers, police officers. How do you deal with that? How do you fuckin' deal with turning up to someone hanging? I've had to regulate my connection and engagement with people because it's really hard if you're not well enough yourself and don't have the capacity to cope.

In Māoridom, and the same in Samoa, there's Te Whare Tapa Whā, the four-wall model of health. Taha wairua, taha hinengaro, taha tinana, taha whānau. Spiritual, mental, physical and family. Those four elements, those four walls, make up a being, and you're in big trouble if you deny one of them. They all need to be in balance. Up till now, mainstream healthcare has not acknowledged the spiritual aspects of health enough, but I think the world's changing; I think we are becoming more holistic and more aware.

One of the skill sets I had to learn, and I think it was something I was born with and had to develop, was listening, man. Listening is such a key thing. And not judging. I think it's the most important gift and tool in the community. I have been to heaps of different conferences and I've watched kids be like, You never listen. You don't get me. You don't understand me. And it's more complex than that, but still. Listening is making people feel heard, which makes them feel safe, comfortable and able to open up to you, able to be vulnerable about the anxieties and things they're going through. Supporting people is its own kaupapa. You try to create experiences where you can affirm people and feel affirmed. I think the key for youth is to be affirmed by their peers, publicly. It's the same with women, men, everyone.

I quit my job recently. I felt the wairua pulling me out. I had a stint in politics last year, which was amazing. I ran for the Māori Party for Christchurch East. This is our first problem as Māori and Pasifika: there is nowhere for us to claim as our own in the city. I have seen Gerry Brownlee's blueprint; there is nothing in the city that is Pacific or Māori. Everywhere you look, it's white. On the council there are 10 people, and they're all white, except for that beautiful man Raf Manji, who ran independently. We don't even have Samoans on senior leadership teams, on council, as lawyers—nothing. Why would our kids aspire to be anyone in this city? Our faces aren't anywhere. That's why I did politics. I just wanted my face on a billboard in the east, so all the kids could say, Hey. I know that guy. He is one of us.

State Cinema

A STAR IS BORN

H-6

08:45 PM   17 2018

State Cinema

A STAR IS BORN

H-6

08:45 PM   17 2018

Not Standing Upright There

Paul Stanley Ward

I've always had a thing for birds. I grew up in Marton. The farming service town's slogan touted it as 'the hub of the Rangitikei', lest it wither in isolation, bypassed by State Highway 1. But it felt like the edge of the world. We used to grip electric fences for a buzz. In the 80s, its youth suicide rate made getting out alive an accomplishment. The war memorial pou remembers the dead, young men who died fighting for the land of milk and honey; generations later, young men die less gloriously as mental health statistics.

The escape offered by flight was seductive—kāhu circled high over the plains—but flight wasn't necessary to the birds' appeal. To this small-town cop's son, it was their freakiness that seduced: birds were my Bowie. On a pig hunt as a teenager, while mates were hooning after the dogs, I was distracted by the miromiro and kārearea, unlikely relics from *Buller's Book of Birds*, now exotic in the plantation pine trees. For me, their evolutionary quirks made them as unique to Aotearoa as the All Blacks. These manu carried stories; they had homegrown mystique. The orange glow of the kāhu's underwing was the scar of Māui's mission to bring back fire from Mahuika.

As much as I loved Ewoks and *E.T.*, I was intrigued by a school lesson on poet Allen Curnow's famous moa.[1] In 1943 Curnow remembered a boyhood encounter in Canterbury Museum with the skeleton of a giant three-metre-tall bird with *The Guinness World Records* stature: 'Not I, some child,

---

1 Allen Curnow, 'Attitudes for a New Zealand Poet (III): The Skeleton of the Great Moa in the Canterbury Museum, Christchurch', in *Collected Poems*, ed. Elizabeth Caffin and Terry Sturm (Auckland: AUP, 2017).

born in a marvellous year . . . will learn the trick of standing upright here.' As an adult at the beginning of the 21st century, I found literal meaning in Curnow's metaphor: I was working in Venice, Los Angeles, and having trouble standing upright there. It wasn't the drive-by shootings. It wasn't even the earthquakes, or the Burning Man parties. It was the concrete.

Out of the blue, I'd passed out twice.

The first time was a hungover Sunday. I'd walked down to Venice Beach for a bodysurf. I dried off on the grass by the roller derby, feeling the sun's warmth on my lids, eying the dreamcatcher spruikers and that rollerblading guitarist from the 90s New Zealand TV ad for chocolate milk (it was like seeing Māui in the flesh).

On standing, I felt my heart hold back a beat. My legs crumpled like a marionette with the strings cut. A skater rolled over to help me up.

I was producing for a Discovery Channel reality TV show. I was in my mid 20s and employed in the entertainment industry. It was a vague box-tick. I felt okay about the show because it was about achieving dreams rather than fetishising human frailty.

The second fade-to-black happened after I'd filmed a story about a kick-boxer from the hood who trained celebrity clients at his Venice gym. The boxer's tele-dream was to build a ring for needy kids in South Central, and we were picking up shots to emphasise the *Rocky* arc. A boxer punched a '1-2-3' combo on a bag. A metallic 'pop pop pop' echoed it outside. Thirty metres away, on the rim of the Venice Circle, a black kid lay on the tarmac. Blood seeped onto the concrete with CGI fluidity.

When released from the police cordon, we drove down to Watts Towers. Outside the police station we filmed the ex-leader of the Crips gang: 'Kids here is lucky to get to your age. Growing up here is like living in a war zone.' On cue, gun shots drummed out blocks away, and squad cars spat from the garage.

Amid the sirens, what seemed to be a large bee hovered above a shrub, like a detail in a Sergio Leone western. Looking closer, I saw it was a hummingbird—my first. Manic wingbeat, honeysucker bill, oil slick in the sun.

That night, I returned to Santa Monica to debrief with my friend Anya, who was ferrying cocktails to stars at Casa Del Mar. Later we watched *21 Grams* and pondered guns, the size of popcorn servings and the weight of the soul. In the car park's concrete geometry I felt woozy trying the door handle of Anya's wide-beamed station wagon. My eyes rolled and my gut lurched. The door took my weight as Outkast shook it like a Polaroid picture on the stereo.

MRIs came back clear, but the spells continued and an apprehension of fainting began to creep into my LA days. The spells piqued my sense of self-control. I had been reared on the Kiwi male Spartan traditions of rugby and rowing. The bookends of our family shelf featured the twin peaks of *Colin Meads: All Black* and *Mark of a Lion: the Story of Charles Upham V.C. and Bar*. As a teenager, I had imported a mail-order weightlifting guide from LA. Wellington's northern suburb garages became Muscle Beach for a trio of teen Mr Universe wannabes. We chugged Body Bulk, loaded shoplifted plates and followed *The Weider System*'s 'no pain, no gain' mantra. Schwarzenegger was our Nietzsche.

Lifting weights, along with car-roof surfing and rutting on clothes lines, was extracurricular to my single-sex boys school education. There, we were indoctrinated into a culture based around academic and sporting achievement. Garter checks, Kipling, mass haka and assembly songs equating sacrifice on the footy field with sacrifice on the battlefield—bizarre in the 90s (the 1990s, not the 1890s). The subtext was entitlement and a moral superiority gained through exertion or will (or your parent being a real estate agent, diplomat or car dealer). As a suburban striver I bought into it and went about accruing the badges: 1st XV rugby, prefect—I was the first person in my family to gain university entrance.

Thus, I was sure my LA spells were physiological. To sweat it out I sat on a rowing machine at Gold's Gym and I went running in Griffith Park, thinking of mountain lions, brain tumours and James Dean. Here there was no risk of fainting—even in the dusty heat—searching for a collision of endorphins and environment to take me out of my body. I didn't know it then but I was running from the hills of Te Whanganui a Tara.

From the edge of the world, Los Angeles was one of a clutch of destinations that Air New Zealand flew to direct, tracing umbilical paths to global centres. Waka conveyed Māori stories to Aotearoa on the great migration from Hawaiki. Most of Pākehā New Zealand's traditional stories are seated on a Gandalf-emblazoned 747 from Hollywood.

During school holidays growing up, daytime soaps like *Santa Barbara* stood in loco parentis. My more sophisticated mates yearned for Manchester or Dunedin on their teenage bedroom CD players; not I. I was 'Born in the USA', stone-washed and into hair metal. Even my father's VHS porn collection was made in LA. (The Vaseline-soft sunlight and Hollywood Hills pools felt . . . intimately familiar.)

Like a classics scholar visiting Rome or Athens, I went on a pilgrimage to the LA intersection where Bruce Willis crashes in *Pulp Fiction*. The song scoring that scene, 'Flowers on the Wall' ('smoking cigarettes and watching Captain Kan-ga-roo . . .') wormed about in my ear. It was the same tune that opened the Kiwi TV classic *A Dog's Show*.

Bleary-eyed in the heat at a Los Feliz market, I picked up a blue 1998 Teen and Miss Barstow Pageant T-shirt and added another spell to my tally. Kiwi struggle in drought: when the ground hardens, their chopstick beaks can't probe to snaffle grubs and worms. I too began to be conscious of walking on hard earth.

This time the doctor skipped the tests and wrote me a prescription: Lexapro. Googling revealed generalised anxiety disorder and depression. Eh? My Type A ego was insulted, and I was unnerved by the possible side effect of suicidal thoughts. But my Angeleno passport was stamped. This was the town of the IMAX, Self-Realization Fellowship, and Scientology. Triumph of the pill.

To supplement the serotonin capsule, I gnawed at a cause so I could fix 'it'. My schoolteacher mum would've asked if I was burning the candle at both ends. Work hours were long, but I was capable and, drive-by excepted, comfortable.

Was 'it' the ecology of denial? LA was built on the edge of the desert and tectonic plates, but the dirt was coated with concrete—even the river runs over concrete—disguised with freeways, fairways and tropical palms. Was 'it' culture shock? But I was enthralled. I went out wide-eyed, scoping the strip malls, waxy industry town and under-the-bridge underworlds, expanding my horizons and all that OE guff.

I didn't know it then, but when I wasn't gawking, I was homesick. Not I, a kāhu or soaring kea, but a half-blind kiwi, squinting under the desert sun's flare.

I was flummoxed by the spells' schedule: I could run for hours with the coyotes in the canyons, but would be felled inside an Ikea display room. Fluorescent lighting was a trigger. Between the high shelving of the Silver Lake 99c store my heart skipped, the sands slipped through the hourglass and I deflated on the lino.

I noted the date on Santa Monica's historic Roy Jones house: 1894. This American city (post Chumash, Tongva, Spanish and Mexican habitation) was younger than Pākehā New Zealand, than Johnsonville or Geraldine. California, like New Zealand, is a new idea. In Griffith Park I saw that the Hollywood sign was just a modest-sized real estate advert.

Laconic Pākehā New Zealand doesn't go in much for myth-making, or for prescription solutions popped out of silver foil. Official selections in a recent flag-change debate were eclipsed by a clip-art kiwi with a laser beaming out of its eye. When it comes to a song to represent us on a marae, we Pākehā males struggle for choices; sports terraces ring with piss-sinking anthem *Bliss*—'forget about the last one, get yourself another'—but without booze we're more uptight than upright. At funerals, eulogisers are praised for keeping it together, for not expressing too much.

This New Zealand emotional economy can be punchy: Christchurch was 'munted' after the 2011 earthquakes. 'Bugger' is deployed in the wake of small-to-medium scale catastrophe. Sam Neill's Uncle Hec in *Hunt for the Wilderpeople* found laughs (and pathos) because he is still recognisable as a Kiwi archetype, the man of few words.

But the flip side? Was munted an apt description of our emotional literacy? Was my body articulating a response to spite its limited vocabulary?

While I was a sensitive student (Drama! Debating!), raised to respect women, my understanding of meaningful relationships with wāhine was a BA in binge-drinking. The Lord's Prayer and Blake's 'Jerusalem' turned out not to be ideal primers for young adulthood at the turn of the millennium. And *The Joy of Sex*, high in my parents' wardrobe, offered few physical pointers to a child of the pre-Pornhub era.

Far from the intricate Fiordland tango of the kākāpō's courtship ritual, dating in Aotearoa is performed when drunk or high, late at night on sports fields, in dank flats or skate bowls. After having sex, you undertake the walk of shame. These furtive couplings—it took years to remember sex—were a foggy introduction to physical intimacy. Other than in the ruck or scrum, I'd barely touched another body. I don't recall hugging my father before I was 21. Mean.

The light being received and passed on in my school's Latin

motto—*lumen accipe et imperti*—was not the light of love or aroha, mindfulness, or even small talk. Girls, who you only met at socials or stared at from a distance at bus stops, were just another thing that we were entitled to as 'col boys'. A result of that entitlement was non-consensual sex. As Roast Busters and the WC Boy controversy confirm, it's just as true 20 years on. 'If you don't take advantage of a drunk girl, you're not a true WC [Wellington College] boy', claimed a Facebook post in 2017.

Aotearoa has long marketed itself as 100% Pure. The untouched brand seems to have been taken literally as a national anti-intimacy instruction. No hongi or hugs here, just a haphephobic trembling beneath an up-and-under kick, as the fear of being wet or gay drops from the sky. Arguably this virginity precludes us from discussing war, colonialism, sex or anxiety. Chur.

Kiwis tend to stereotype Americans as loud, as false or inauthentic, but in relation to what? Being staunch? Dumb silence?

As an inheritor of that bottled-up 'she'll be right' therapy tradition, I kept my falling down secret from my LA amigos, remembering the five Ps of my PE teacher: Pride in Presentation Produces Perfection in Performance. A Kiwi import that was doing a better job of standing upright here was the pōhutukawa, whose roots were cracking up Santa Monica's sidewalks. Before I cracked the pavement again, my visa expired and I found myself across the other side of the Pacific, back in Wellington.

It was midwinter. Unemployed. Girlfriend wanted kids. The anxiety attacks (that's what they were, defined retrospectively) had been replaced with a young man's fear of commitment. Wellington was middle-of-the-road Middle Earth, with denizens sheltering in wooden villas from the southerly. I had returned home with meagre expectations. Bugger.

I ran to the hills. Through the suburbs and the gorse's stigmata, up to the wind turbine. Nothing to think about, just the bullish grunt to get above it all and watch clouds fast-forward over the harbour. In Wellington the wind redistributes trampolines and plastic bags like a celestial leaf blower.

The blustery rain was an embrace. Coming down Raroa Road, I stooped to tie my laces and looked down over the quaint cold town of Aro Valley. As I was pondering where the bad air gets dumped by Tāwhirimātea, bits of it pitter-pattered on my cap.

I looked up into the branches of a gum tree. It wasn't rain, but bark chip. The axeman was a kākā.

I was baffled. I'd never seen the bush parrot in the city. As a kid I'd nagged my parents to take me to far-flung sanctuaries to see kākā, kōkako, tawaki and kiwi.

I felt a kinship with the birds, with their quixotic right to exist. Like Morrissey or Bruce, Auel or Prince, they offered a wild salve to suburbia. Ecologists consider them to be deeply endemic. In Māori myth they were born from Rangi and Papa's interrupted love-making, imagined with rare sensuality. In Don Merton's estimation they're our Tower of London, our Arc de Triomphe, our pyramids. But they're also primitivists, struggling with the rat race. Introduced predators and habitat loss have rendered many of them extinct or exiled to islands.

So how did the 21st-century kākā get to be here, in the Aro gum? The birds of Wellington city that I knew as a student in the 90s were introduced pigeons and sparrows, emblems of any city anywhere, mangy birds of the eaves and underpasses.

But kākā? Prehistoric punks in supplejack rafters, sure, but not road warriors. Its only Wellington contemporaries were stuffed in a museum with Curnow's moa. I took a key from my shorts and rubbed it between my fingers. The big rufous parrot hopped down the branch. With a push and flap it was on my forearm, trying to prise the key. I was gobsmacked—touched.

Hallelujah, St Francis. But this kākā was not mine to bid. Bored, it tilted its head. With a wheelspin it was away across the valley, flashing its underwing, a blaze of orange in the dawn.

The Lexapro and sidewalk body-slams scudded back across the Pacific. Chill. I'd be all right here. I ran home past the sleepers, not fretful at all. The parrot whispered the same secret as that moa. I forgot about Chinatown and California girls and ran towards something bigger than me. Towards Lucy, and Estella and Sylvie (born in water). I recognised a flock of unreconstructed southern souls working on garage projects, salt-blasted on the coast with their collars up, leaning into the wind with shining secrets hidden under their wings.

I went running in Griffith Park thinking of mountain lions, brain tumours and James Dean. I didn't know it then but I was running from the hills of Te Whanganui a Tara. The kākā told me so when I got home. I, born on the not-especially-marvellous cusp of Gen Y, was shown the trick of standing upright here.

The Beginning

Aimie Cronin

I am 39 weeks and two days pregnant. As I waddled into the post office yesterday, the nice man behind the counter took one look at me and said, 'You should not be out like this. Stay inside the house until baby comes.' Three people stopped and stared as I walked to my car. 'When are you due?' one called out from way across the car park. 'Any day now,' I said. She tilted her head as if to say, Holy hell! 'Yeah, you are,' she said. I feel in equal parts like beauty at its highest and a big fat lump.

For months I have been looking at expiry dates with no interest other than their proximity to the date I am due to give birth to my first baby. I tell my husband, and he decides that a bottle of milk holds the ultimate expiry date: that when those bold numbers assert themselves from the fridge with a date that matches ours, it will mean this is officially happening, like a stamp landing on a passport when you arrive in a new country.

Last week we visited the supermarket and I reached down the back for the new milks, and there it was. 'We don't need milk,' my husband said. I looked at him in disbelief, pointing to the date. 'It's a keepsake!'

At home, I can't stop opening the fridge to stare at the bottle. I take a photo of it, snapchatting it to friends with the date circled and the baby emoji and a shocked faced emoji and a heart emoji. They respond with the clapping hands emoji, the heart emoji, the emoji where the yellow face is laughing till it cries. I engage with all of these interactions in good humour, but somewhere inside I feel a shock bordering on panic that the day of the milk expiry match has arrived, and sometime soon an *actual* baby will arrive as well.

I also partake in the euphoric and frightening exercise of measuring this time in 'last's. I think, This could be the last time I wash my hair before the baby comes, the last time I eat Dan Dan noodles, the last time I have to cut my toenails, the last time I change the sheets, the last time I buy something online, the last time I see Everywhere Man as I drive down the street. When my friends say goodbye, they say, This could be the last time I see you before you have a baby! And I shut the door and cannot for the life of me believe it's real.

For four years, my husband and I wanted nothing more than a baby, and in those years we learned that no matter how much you want something, or how much you try, it might happen, but there's a chance it won't. I grew up in the age of the Aha! moment, watching people who wrote books like *The Secret* sit on Oprah's couch and tell her to put out to the universe what she wants to get back. Our whole lives we are taught that if we work hard enough, we will get what we want. How do we reconcile that with the bleak prospect of infertility?

My friend said recently that pregnancy is a constant state of mild to elevated panic, and indeed I feel like this: mild panic with every ache and pain, elevated panic at the eight ultrasounds we've elected this time around, where I still can't look at the screen and see anything but all my life and happiness hanging in the balance of the black and white blobs moving around, looking ominous.

'I get really anxious with scans, just so you know,' I tell the sonographers each time. They smile and are probably thinking, *Great*.

'Is this your first pregnancy?' they ask.

'No, my third, but the other two didn't happen,' I say.

'Okay,' they say. 'Let's have a look.'

Seconds pass. 'Is everything okay?' I ask it over and over.

My fear of scans began with the first miscarriage. I look back to that one and think about how optimistic I was, how much I took it for granted that everything would be okay, how completely unexpected the news was, despite the signs I picked over in the years that followed. The first time the sonographer said, 'I'm sorry, this is not a viable pregnancy', it felt like walking into the shade. I lost a kind of innocence about the way life would unfold before me. I remember the scanning rod was still inside me and she was shifting it around, frowning into the monitor for slow minutes, taking stills as I lay there, sentenced to the bed, trying to contain my panic. I had never in my life felt so desperate and frozen all at once. I remember my husband's hand tightening on my arm and, most of all, a black hole on the screen that now, even four years later, I have to distract myself from thinking about. These things change you.

When I fell pregnant the second time, my dog sat still as I cried into her fur, tears of grief and joy. When I told people, I felt self-conscious, choked by happiness, like I was opening a gift in front of them and had to try and convey my gratitude. I couldn't match my words to what was happening in my heart. As the weeks passed, no bleeding, no pain, none of the grim symptoms you read about, I slowly began to let myself relax and discuss the possibility of having a baby with my husband. I was annoyed at him for holding back. 'Just let yourself feel joy,' I said, and each day I felt a little more entitled to claim that what was happening was real. I thought about the black hole from the last ultrasound and there were times when I could make sense of it like a realistic person. I made my husband follow me into conversations about our new life, and we sounded awkward at first, but soon we got so good at dreaming about it. Will our house be warm enough, we whispered to each other, where will it sleep, will the dog be jealous, what do we need, what will we call it? And we gave it a nickname, as you do. At night my husband let his hands smooth over my stomach and sometimes he said goodnight to it and they were among the sweetest moments of my life.

I never felt the first two kick. We lost the second at 15 weeks, just as I was about to show. 'There was a bump,' I cried to my husband after. 'There wasn't,' he says, running his hands through my hair. 'There wasn't.'

Now, nothing settles my anxiety like the feel of this baby kicking. He kicks, 'I'm alive!', and I can carry on living too. He sleeps, and I worry, and my husband and I set the timer and hold my stomach, waiting for him as I try and stay sane. Sometimes at night I think about worse things that may happen to us, and everything we have been through feels like a warning. To love more than this and risk loss is a frightening thing. I shake my husband awake one night, hysterical, to tell him he needs to go to the doctor for a check-up. Chaos threatens, and it's so deep down, at the thought I might ever lose them.

A few months into this pregnancy, I visit a counsellor about my fear of the scans.

'But you're going to them all, you're showing up?' she asks.

I say that I am.

'Acknowledge that,' she says. 'Be kinder to yourself.'

Perhaps it's a sign of progression that I can see myself crashing towards panic and that sometimes I swerve and miss it, just. Other times, I'm all in. By the time my husband gets home from work I am convinced our unborn child is in perilous danger because of half an interview I caught on national radio about bog water—we don't even use bog water—or the bag of lettuce that has been recalled from the supermarket, or the cheese I didn't check at a restaurant. 'What if I poison him?' I say. 'What if I fall over and hit my belly? What if I roll onto my back in the night and he can't breathe?' My husband settles me each time with the same line, as calming as an old song. 'You're well, I'm well, the baby is well,' he says. On we go.

There is a comfort in knowing that time has its way with pain. That eventually the panic dulls because life overrides it. In the weeks following the loss of our second baby, we slowly allowed ourselves to become distracted by everyday things, spending hours with the laptop sitting between us, watching reruns of *Friends*, eating mashed potatoes smothered in salt, picking feijoas in our dressing gowns from beneath the tree out front. My favourite part of the day was going for long drives, looking on at the monotony oozing out of those tidy, middle-class neighbourhoods. I felt calm watching people at their dullest, seeing lights on through netted curtains and the TV playing. One day the sun hit the park when we were walking and I noticed beauty. Our dog ran to the only roped-off corner and pooed; we looked around, embarrassed, then laughed at her rebellion. There was a reassurance in those moments, that life wanders along and is mostly gentle. I pulled flowers from the bouquets we were sent and dotted them around the house in jars so that everywhere we went there were reminders that we are loved, we are loved, we are loved, we are loved. We ate lemon biscuits, hand-delivered by my mum, and saw her little face that wished nothing but good things for us. The anxiety lessened its ringing in my ears. Enough to try again, knowing that no matter how much you want something, or how much you try, it might happen, but there's a chance it won't.

I promised each and every unknown god that my worry would disappear the minute I got pregnant, but I should have known better. Even though I say I will be calmer when he's born—through infancy, childhood, adolescence, adulthood—there will be times, I'm sure, when I will lose all rational thought. But as I write this, only days away from holding him, all that matters to me is that he's almost here, and my arms tingle at the prospect of it.

This week at the supermarket, a woman stocking shelves sees me and drops a box full of canned fruit. 'I got distracted by your stomach!'

A stranger walks past and says, 'Good luck.'

I get to the milk and the expiry date is a week past my due date.

MOTUEKA NEW ZEALAND

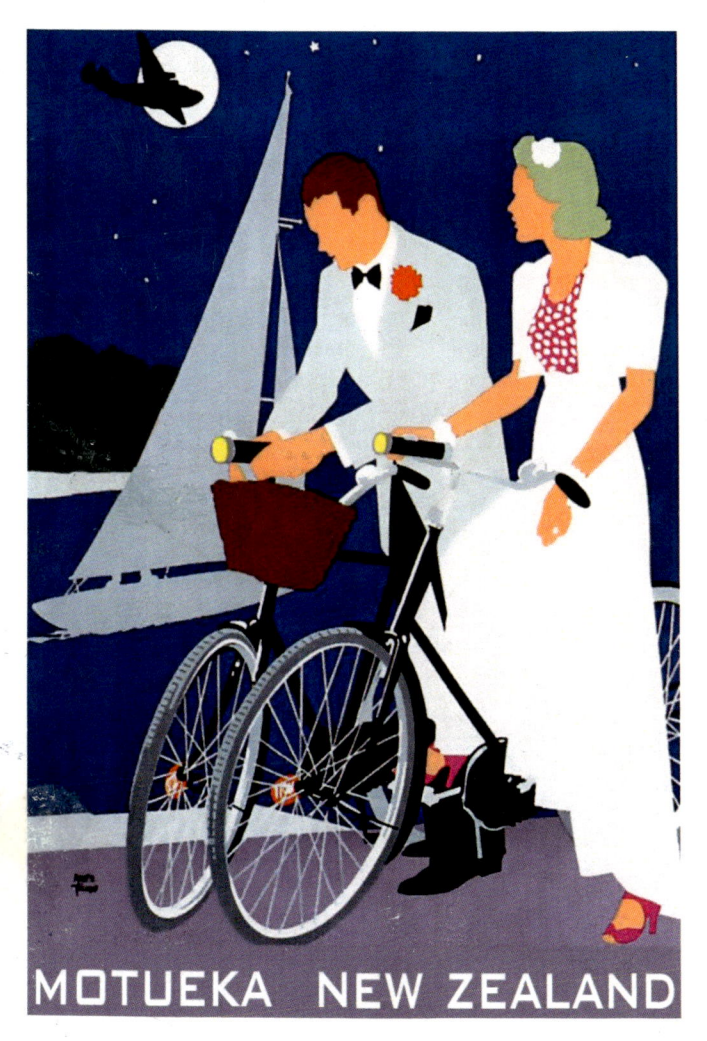

SST02MOTUP

Printed on **FUJI XEROX** Colour eXpressions Silk 300gm card.

NZ ART CARDS

I smile and my heart quickens, but only a little. By the time we reach the new milk expiry date, I will be home with an actual baby. Christ! A 'what if' creeps in, then another. I catch myself, just in time. I place a hand on my stomach and feel the thing I wanted more than anything and now cannot believe I actually have. Sure enough, somewhere inside my busy head, there is joy to be visualised, too. I picture a healthy baby, wrapped tight in his little sleeping basket. I picture myself, checking on him in the night, holding him in my arms. I picture him, peeping out from his capsule as I wander through the supermarket.

In a Scorched Room

Michelle Langstone

It's a fever you catch. It's a heat that ignites in the closest cells in the absolute heart of you and bursts into flames, incinerating every atom in a second. It's the kind of heat that, a hundred-odd years ago, prompted people to exchange cautionary glances and cross themselves when they left the room, murmuring softly under their breath about funeral arrangements. It's a fever nobody should withstand, and yet it comes every time, that wall of heat, and I am still here.

Once I took all my clothes off in a bathroom stall and lay down on the cool tiles, just to try to put the fire out. I rested my face on my folded blue jeans, because inside the furnace I still had the presence of mind to consider germs, even if this was my demise: death by nerves on a cold toilet floor, burning alive in the middle of winter at a restaurant in Mt Eden.

When I was small, I had a grave fear of being misunderstood. I remember writing cards to my parents and drawing hearts all over the cardboard, telling them how much I loved them. Dozens of cards, just in case they forgot.

After my father was diagnosed with cancer we cleared the house of years of clutter, and I found manila folders full of my school things in the cupboard—reports and notebooks and art. Tucked among them were the cards I'd made for my mother and father. One of them apologised profusely for doing things wrong and reiterated my love, over and over, every alphabet letter a different felt-tip pen colour. I felt sad when I saw that card. Sad that someone so small should be worried already, anxious that love might run out. My parents have always loved me like I was a hot air balloon; I am full of their love and elevated by it.

Even as a child, I imagined bursting into flames mid-air. Lying under a gooseberry bush with my sister, popping the sour fruit from their papery skins with an ear out for the neighbours, whose bush we were robbing, I felt my body run quick like an electric current. Even then I could feel that the tension was disproportionate—they'd said we could help ourselves, and the sneaking was a game, but I could not match my feelings with my sister's gleeful excitement. I got so hot I thought I would faint, or set fire to the bush and the house, and then the whole street would burn, and everyone would know it was me, the fire-raiser.

The arc of my youth was a punctured bow. Many moments of happiness, absolutely, but many moments of hot anxiousness and tight palpitation. School became more and more difficult as I tried to navigate friendships under the strain of shyness and nerves. Every single morning I would shout and fight to try and get out of going. I got so anxious I could bring on a fever, which proved helpful in the sick bay on days when it got too much and I just needed to go home.

Much of my 20s were a haze of smoke and embers. I remember nothing of an industry awards ceremony—in a gown, in make-up, in the midst of celebration—save the white linen napkin in my hands, and the way I lined the seam of its hem along the line of my palm, and how I looked at it again and again, like a touchstone, to draw me back into the room. The napkin white, my dress white, my palm on fire, my insides blazing. I had the sense of being absolutely wrong: in the wrong place, in the wrong time, in the wrong body.

At some point, at a loose end and feeling hollowed by fire, I reached out to a bird rescue centre and asked if I could volunteer. I was alone in a big house in Bronte, Sydney, and had just received a recriminatory email from an ex-boyfriend that had sent me into absolute panic. It was cool outside, rainy and wet, and it was hot inside, everything molten and running away from me.

On that day, a New Zealand musician I followed on Twitter had retweeted a photo of a bird being cared for at a rescue centre in Auckland. I looked through their account, enchanted by all the birds in various states of wellness. It reminded me of the times after storms when my sister and I would climb over the fence at the end of our road and search the farmland for nests and baby birds that had been shaken from the trees by the wind. We cared for so many as children, never with great success, but with a huge sense of importance and tenderness.

I turned up several weeks later, on a wet Sunday morning in autumn, to a place near Green Bay in Auckland, to put myself to work. The two-storey house was perched on a hill up a wide driveway, and was home to a woman who dedicated all her time to caring for birds. A ranch slider door downstairs dragged open to a room crammed with cages and cacophony. You've never been greeted the way a room full of birds greets you when you're first to arrive in the morning. It's a rowdy, joyful thing—some birds are delighted, some are very cross and muttering in their half-asleep state, and many are just pleased that something is happening.

In the beginning it was my job to care for the caged birds. I learned to clean their cages by hand, to change the paper or soft towels that lined their boxes and crates and metal houses, to wash their food and water bowls in hot water, to bring them little treats of fruit, or a toy to play with, and to tend to their specific needs.

They were many parrots. Some had been abandoned. One was surrendered after his owner passed away; others had escaped their homes and were waiting to see if anyone missed them. Some had been bought for ceremonies and just let go into the sky in a flash of colour, lost in a world they had never met, a world that held no shape or safety for them. Many of the birds were anxious, their sharp eyes on me and their beaks ready to bite my new hands.

One lorikeet had deformed feet with claws that curled over, which made it hard for him to perch. His cage was full of platforms made from donated gauze sheets with plastic backing, which covered the metal wire so that his feet wouldn't get caught. Whenever I opened the cage, this little bird would hop onto my hand and loll about, not quite standing, not quite keeled over, but sort of stumbling on his misshapen feet. His eyes were keenly bright, and he watched me intently as I made adjustments to his home. When I would move to put him back he would resist, because he liked my hand, and he liked my company, and it would always take a moment to get him settled and reacquainted with his ladder and his platforms, as if he had briefly forgotten where he lived.

There were cages with native birds, too. A juvenile ruru turned his beacon eyes on me when I lifted a tea towel to look in at him in the dark. An orphaned baby pūkeko was in an incubator, keeping warm while he grew his tiny indigo feathers. A pīwakawaka missing feathers from his fan tail hopped back and forth on a beam, impatient. Every bird needed to be cared for by hand.

We had ducks at Bird Rescue, picked up in parks because they were gravely ill with botulism, most likely from eating mouldy bread thrown by well-meaning people. When a bird has botulism its muscles get very floppy and it cannot hold up its head. A duck with botulism is a duck in absolute despair. It was my job to bathe them in the outdoor sink, to keep them clean and comfortable. I would lower them gently into the water and rest their heads on a rolled up towel that kept their beaks and nostrils above water, or I would lay their soft heads over my forearm. There, in the cool water, their tired bodies would float and sway while they closed their eyes and seemed to drift away inside. Sometimes the water would revive one of them enough that they would be tempted by a piece of fresh white bread roll. Those were very good days for my heart.

Eventually I graduated from the indoor birds and began to include some outdoor birds in my care routine. Outside around the property there were huge wooden and metal cages for birds who needed more space. There was a 'swoop coop' for a clutch of kōtare babies who were learning how to fly. Their croaking radio static commentary would begin the moment they saw me approach the cage, carrying the smushed-up, stinking food I had prepared for them, and they'd watch me from beneath their baby feathers and flat heads with suspicion. They were so small and so misshapen, it was hard to imagine the sleek creatures they would become. As they grew braver, they taught each other to fly. One bold bird would tumble from the perch and catch itself and land somehow on the other side of the cage looking surprised, and the others would follow.

Nearby, one of their relatives, a kookaburra, had an old wooden cage to himself. It was taller than I was, the front entirely wrapped in mesh, with a little door to the side for giving him food and changing his water. He'd sit on that branch, alone, ruffled and seeming confused, and I would walk by and meet his gaze and think, *Same*.

When I met those birds, my experience of anxiety started to change. They were so much more exposed than I was, and caring for them made me feel stronger. It lifted me, being able to help. I have always been good in a crisis, so long as it belonged to someone else. Over time I discovered that in protecting and nurturing these animals, I was somehow protecting and nurturing myself.

Weeks passed, and a mild autumn let go into a heavy, cold winter. My hands were red raw from the scalding water and soap of clean cages. Battle-weary seabirds began to arrive at the centre, their wings askew, their bellies empty and their internal compasses swinging wildly in disorientation.

A fisherman turned up one morning carrying a box that

was thumping and swaying in his hands. He'd found a gannet in trouble out on the rocks. We kept him quiet so he could recover, in an opaque white box by the ranch slider door. The lid was made of mesh, and as I passed by I could see him, sitting very still in a corner. Even standing at full height he would not have been able to glimpse the wild he had come from. The lines along the sides of his beak looked like instructions for making paper planes, and he smelled like his home. He was a fishy, salty, unhappy wildling. I could feel his panic whenever someone moved past his cage; I could discern that anxious jolt through my own skin, as if my proximity was a conduit for transference. That gannet and I had the same urge to run, and in him I recognised the leaps and jumps of nerves that mark an anxious spirit. He was out of place, and so was I. I don't know why that brought me comfort, but it did. He waited it out in his cramped quarters. He got stronger and sleeker and stroppier, and then he was set free. I cried when I came to work and found that he was gone. I cried in triumph and a kind of blazing fierce rage because he had endured and had been rewarded. He taught me something, that bird. I could hold on, and after the fire, there would be a new landscape.

I couldn't stay at Bird Rescue forever. Work took me to other places; Sundays became filled with other things. The need to protect and nurture did not leave me, though. In Sydney I looked after a little stray cat, fattened her up and found her a home. I left water out on my balcony for the birds and possums in the high summer, and spied on them through the bathroom window when they came for a drink. Some days I would just move snails and worms into safer places when they'd used the footpaths as motorways after rain. Tiny things, but acts that refocussed my thoughts outside of myself.

I have learned to nurture the fragile life that is closest to me. In the middle of a round of radiation treatment, when Dad's body was starting to break and he shook violently with convulsions, I wrapped my whole self around him and held him until it passed. We lay on the bed in our pyjamas—a tangle of bathrobes and flannel—and I didn't let go until it subsided. I heard Time get his coat and search for his keys, and let himself out. Everything stood still. I told my dad to hold on, and I told him he was brave and was doing a good job, and I told him that I loved him. It was one of the saddest moments I had with Dad around that time, and one of the most tender, but there was no panic in it. I felt the flood of a tide come surging through my body, cooling the heat down so entirely, that for the first time in my life, it seemed as if my insides forgot they were a tinderbox at all.

I don't think the 'why' of anxiety matters to me anymore. I know that it comes when I feel I can't communicate or I am not understood, so I try to speak bravely, I say how I feel and I ask for what I need. And then I look outwards to see if there is anyone else I can help. At times the heat starts to return, but more slowly now—like an old element on a stove that resists a little as you turn the knob, warming reluctantly. What matters is how I move it, and where I allow my focus to land. When I manage it right, like that gannet, I can wait it out and be free again. When I manage it right, I no longer land in a scorched room.

Dream Selves

Kirsten McDougall

> Intellectual curiosity about one's own illness is certainly born of a desire for mastery. If I couldn't cure myself, perhaps I could at least begin to understand myself.
> —Siri Hustvedt[1]

I climb the steps to her office, practising my opening gambit like an actor approaching an audition. I am fit but by the time I reach the top of the steps to knock on her door I'm breathless. I knock three times and she opens the door with her wide smile and says, *Come in*. That is all she says, even once I am seated. Her silence is a part of the therapy because she will never tell me what to do. This silence is excruciating for me.

Over the past few months on a Wednesday afternoon I've had a regular appointment with this wide-smiling woman, my therapist. That word—*therapist*—is one I used to shudder at. As I saw it, therapy was a middle-class indulgence, something for people with fragile egos who needed to blame others for their own failings. That was before depression and anxiety dragged me into a tar pit, filling my lungs so that when I ran, as I have done for years to get ahead of my worries and self-loathing, I could no longer breathe. I took myself to the doctor, who prescribed antidepressants and clonazepam for anxiety attacks. The antidepressants pulled me out of the tar pit, but no pill can cure sadness.

Inside the office my therapist takes my coat. We sit down. All of this is done in silence. I have told her how much silence

---

[1] Siri Hustvedt, *The Shaking Woman or a History of My Nerves* (London, UK: Sceptre, 2011), 6.

threatens me, how I have a need to fill it with chatter. Her silence makes me want to shout and kick the furniture then fall down in a sweaty weeping heap. I think I've told her this. Inside the room it's hard for me to remember what I have and haven't said. My memory, when it comes to my emotions, has always been a bit faulty. This concerns me, because I've read that we secure our memories of an event when that event connects strongly to our emotions. If my memory is so patchy, what does this say about how I connect? Sometimes, when I try to remember parts of my own life, I feel as though it is a dream. Perhaps this is how the past exists for many of us, as an accumulating dream. The present moment is informed by the mood of the dream, just as our morning moods are sometimes swayed by our most vivid of sleep-time dreams. It is now widely believed in neuroscience that a memory is not a master copy of an event; what we recall is the memory from the previous time we summoned it. This goes some way towards explaining the unreliability of police witnesses, because our imaginations, which are crucial for memory formation, add and subtract detail in each retelling. The stories we tell about ourselves, our autobiographies, change as we learn more, and our perspectives change. This knowledge soothes my sense that my memories often feel partly fictional, with me a vague dream figure. However, it does not alleviate my concept of myself as an ephemeral thing, a shapeshifter covered in bones and skin—not yet.

Slowly, my therapist has gained my trust and I've told her things about me. Through listening to me talk she has learned about my harsh self-judgement, self-loathing, shame, deep sadness and my sense that, underneath all the faces I've constructed for the outside world, I am nothing. It was she who named my breathlessness 'anxiety'. 'But I'm not an anxious person,' I told her. My image of anxiety was someone housebound and sweaty with nerves, an idea probably received from movies and crappy popular science articles published in weekend papers. Such caricatures of anxiety do nothing to aid our understanding of it. Still, it's hard to understand feelings I rarely acknowledge; I guard my shame and self-loathing like a border terrier patrols a fenceline—let no one enter, not even myself. People have told me I come across as a confident person. I've even been called 'authoritative'. I don't understand this massive gap between what I feel myself to be and what others perceive. Which is the true self? What I call denial—because 'I am not an anxious person'—my therapist calls anxiety. Do these words matter? How precisely must we name these parts of ourselves in order to comprehend them?

It was my therapist who introduced me to the phrase 'the unthought known', which led me to read Christopher Bollas's seminal text *The Shadow of the Object*.[2] I grabbed hold of the term because it spoke to something I could not articulate about myself. The basic sense of the term 'unthought known' in psychoanalysis is a description of those things we know to be true without having consciously thought or cognitively processed them. Bollas says that our unthought knowledge comes from a time when we were preverbal babes in arms, having preverbal, preconscious experiences. We recognise what is in front of us but are unable to bring it to conscious thought. The unthought known can determine our behaviour as older children and adults, behaviours which come to us automatically, and of which we may not understand the root cause. As babies we absorb those experiences we have with our early caregivers, usually and primarily with our mothers. I remember watching my own babies, holding them close to my face and smiling, talking and cooing to them, as they slowly learned to copy me.

As a child I often felt guilty of doing something wrong. This is a difficult paragraph for me to write—as I read over it and

---

2   Christopher Bollas, *The Shadow of the Object: Psychoanalysis of the Unknown Thought* (New York, NY: Columbia University Press, 2017; anniversary edition).

attempt to refine it I'm aware that I fear being judged. My mother raised my sister and me by herself from when I was age four, my sister two. She was strict, but not unloving. I can understand now how the rules she had us live by—so many rules, it seemed to me at the time, with little room to move around them—were probably to give her some sense of control in a life where it must have felt like any control she had over her life had been stripped away when my father left. Her days would have been full, raising us, and I know we had little money. I understand now how she must have felt she was always at full capacity, that anything difficult or out of the ordinary was too much. I myself have a tendency to see red when my kids do something to interrupt the steady flow of the day—like come into the house dripping seawater and sand everywhere. It is only when I stop and say to myself, 'It's only water, it's only sand,' that I can chill out about it. My youngest son says, 'You're always so angry with us,' but I don't think I am. Perhaps my own mother didn't think she was either. I grew up feeling like I wasn't understood or seen for who I sensed myself to be. There is still a large gap between my mother and myself that I struggle to understand. I can only put it down to the difficulties she had when I was a child, trauma in her own life and a distinct difference in our personalities. I cannot say this is why I developed anxiety and depression, but I do believe it is a part of my sense of myself as being insubstantial, with a past as thin as cloud.

Desperate anxiety—the type that has left me unable to breathe, that has shut my body down because the thoughts I had about myself were so unbearable—is interlinked with my depression. I do not know if this is the case for all people, but it is the case for me. The best way I can explain my own anxiety is that there is a boulder rolling down a hill towards me and I'm unable to move out the way. All I can do is raise my arms and shout, 'No no no no!' The 'no' is my anxiety and the boulder is my ball of grief, the denial of how I really feel. The deep grief

I've felt for a lot of my life, of my own sense of not being enough and not being anything to begin with, has been a slow drip on the foundation stone of my core, wearing me down until there was nothing much at my core, nothing to speak of.

It bothers me that I cannot see inside my own body when I get a pain in my calf muscle or a stomach complaint, because I've always thought that if I could look inside my own unconscious, I might be able to understand my problem and fix it. Just as a brain surgeon must precisely target the tissue causing a patient's problem, I too feel that my own psychological surgery must be sober, educated and experienced; and I cannot do it alone. I like this surgery metaphor because I believe we cannot grow in understanding without some painful transformation. Yes, it hurts, but it serves a purpose. I believe an attempt at precision when working to understand ourselves better is important; I am also profoundly aware of my own limitations and blindnesses when it comes to understanding myself, my world and others. I feel like my centre for comprehension (is this my brain, heart, stomach, or all three?) is covered in a layer of blubber, insulating me from true understanding.

Recently I've been reading about the brain–gut connection, how we have neurons in our gut lining and the condition of our gut can affect our moods. Throughout my life I've tried out concepts to help cure myself. Meditation, drinking, running, abstemiousness, veganism, low-fat, full-fat, no sugars, no carbs, poetry, astrology, gardening, fermentation, full-time parenting, full-time working; this is a partial list of my failures. The only ones that really stuck were drinking and sauerkraut. None of them has provided an answer. None of them has helped me understand who I am.

My therapist tells me that I intellectualise my experiences. I nod enthusiastically and take it as a compliment, until I realise that it isn't. What she is trying to get me to do is *feel* my experiences. I explain to her that understanding what goes on in my head and my body—researching neuroscience, psychoanalysis and trauma theory—helps me to hold myself up like an object and examine it. Without this, I feel powerless. I crave self-knowledge and understanding because I want my unthought known to become a thought known. This will always be a struggle for me, though, because whenever we discuss something that raises a strong emotion she says, 'Just sit with that feeling,' and I can't. I find it almost impossible to do. When she first suggested that I sit with my feelings I didn't understand what she meant; it was a concept so foreign to me. For most of my life I've run from how I feel because I fear that feelings will make me too hungry, too sad, too much to handle—the 'oversensitive child'. I have developed a set of sophisticated avoidance skills which keep me from drawing my feelings about past events to the fore, although it is now something I practise. The process has made me consider what it means to try to comprehend and explain myself. When my therapist asks me how an event in my life felt, I have been able to think about it and say 'I felt sad' or 'I felt angry', but whether speaking aloud those phrases renders those feelings real for me is uncertain from session to session. What a blunt tool a simple descriptive phrase such as 'I felt sad' is, so often inadequate to the task. I'm describing a child's scribble, a gathering cloud in the sky.

Language is supposed to enable us to make our conscious selves tangible and open to understanding; words are supposed to give access to our emotions and thoughts, to shape what otherwise might seem an indefinable mass of existence. Without language to shape and describe it, can a conscious mind be said to exist? By signalling an emotion with a referent name, even if this signalling is done only in private to ourselves, we are acknowledging it lives and that we know it lives. But a single word or even a complex sentence often won't be able to express the contradictions and complexity of feelings that humans are capable of holding in themselves at once. What's fabulous and weird is how we've invented ways to convey complexity; humans use figurative language to sharpen our tools. We use metaphor, simile, symbol, parable or allegory to explain things to ourselves. We use abstraction to tell the truth. It's as though we must pass ourselves back and forth through Google Translate in order for our experiences to become digestible to our own intelligences.

In Bessel van der Kolk's brilliant book on trauma, *The Body Keeps the Score*, he writes, 'the language center of the brain is about as far removed from the center for experiencing one's self as is geographically possible. Most of us are better at describing someone else than we are at describing ourselves.'[3] Perhaps this is why we value metaphor so much—because it bridges language and our experiential self. Maybe this is why art exists. Recently, watching footage of young queer South Aucklanders vogue, I thought their vogue battles expressed anger, beauty, fierceness, hope and complexity far more effectively than words ever could.

I am obliged to perform in complete darkness
operations of great delicacy
on my self.[4]

I fell in love with Berryman's *Dream Songs* when I first discovered them many years ago. A deeply distressed man, Berryman was an alcoholic who eventually committed suicide. *Dream Songs* speak to me of the many selves we hold within our one body—our crazy, angry, bored and sad selves.

3   Bessel van der Kolk, *The Body Keeps the Score: Brain, Mind, and Body in the Healing of Trauma* (New York, NY: Viking, 2014), 237.
4   John Berryman, '67' from *The Dream Songs* (New York: Farrar, Straus & Giroux, 1969).

The best poems imitate our partial understandings of ourselves at the same time as drawing a precise image, making a sound, issuing an utterance that feels within our grasp of knowledge. Wallace Stevens said poetry should 'resist the intelligence, almost successfully'. Reading Berryman, reading Manhire, reading Hopkins, I feel like I am being whispered some secret understanding in a language I used to know. Sometimes the closest I've come to understanding myself has been through reading a poem, watching dance, listening to music. Poetry, movement, music—all tools of communication, but what is it that we're trying to communicate? I believe it is our dream selves, those under-articulated, hidden and misunderstood parts of ourselves that don't get noticed as we would like, that never behave as they should, that we are ashamed of and that do not conform to the rules that our culture lays down for us. We are, after all, finite animals capable of dreaming infinity. There have been times in my life when the concept of infinity has almost melted my brain, when the idea that things could go on and on has seemed cruel and alien. And then there are those golden days when infinity seems like hope, because things *can* go on and on and *anything* is possible—if we look after ourselves and one another.

Anxiety sucks. It's one of the worst feelings I've ever felt, apart from when I had suspected meningitis and the doctor gave me a spinal tap. Sometimes I wonder—if I could take a pill to rid myself of anxiety and depression, would I? I'm not sure I would, because I am starting to get the idea that these two monsters have helped me in some way, that they've forced me to face the gap I've ignored for most of my life, between how I feel and how I act. I'm at the point where the gaps no longer scare me, but make me curious about myself, and about gaps in others. I can't be so sanguine about them all the time, but these monsters are *my* monsters, and some days I almost feel affectionate towards them.

My therapist's office is high on a hill facing the harbour. Through the hours I've spent weeping and talking with her, I have watched planes come in to land, clouds cast city-sized shadows over the buildings, kākā, tūī and seagulls ride currents in the wind—all this, over and above. The city astounds me. The birds astound me. How can messy humans, who hurt and abuse one another, who have no idea where to begin healing themselves, build such places? Where do we find the energy for such creation?

On Citalopram

Anthony Byrt

Capitalism is what is left when beliefs have collapsed at the level of ritual or symbolic elaboration, and all that is left is the consumer-spectator, trudging through the ruins and the relics.
—Mark Fisher[1]

The video for Danny Brown's 2016 song 'Pneumonia' opens with four quick cuts. In the first, we see chains being pulled upwards. Then, a flash of Brown himself lying on tarmac. After that, the chains again. Finally, Brown's face, upside down, his head swollen with the pressure of rushing blood, droplets of sweat running up his face. Behind him, a bank of old TVs throws pale light. Brown's eyes open: a gasp of air, a terrified look.

The chains, we realise seconds later in the glare of the overhead lights, have hauled Brown up from the tarmac. He's suspended in midair, part marionette, part lynching victim. We don't know who did it—there's no torturer visible, nor even the frame the chains are mounted on: a midnight carpark racking carried out by invisible hands.

From the opening hook onwards ('Made 30 bands in 30 minutes / Before I count it I done damn near spent it'),[2] the song is as immobilising as the chains. It's a desperate story of drug use, self-degradation and anonymous sex, all of it underpinned by Brown's commercial success: his house in the Michigan suburbs, his designer clothes, sex and drugs on demand. It's the

---

[1] *Capitalist Realism: Is There No Alternative?* (John Hunt Publishing, 2009), 4.
[2] 'Pneumonia', track 9 on Danny Brown, *Atrocity Exhibition*, Copper Top / Red Bull, 2016.

hip-hop version of the American Dream, the kind of lifestyle celebrated by rappers of the 90s and early 2000s. Why, then, is Brown so fucking depressed about it?

We're given some clues, such as archival footage of Ronald Reagan and George H.W. Bush celebrating at Republican National Conventions; elated white folk waving American flags at them; a young man holding up a sign that reads 'Youth ♥ Reagan'; Barbara Bush smiling with her strings of pearls and hard-set Thatcher hair. All of this is spliced with shots of Brown behind a lectern in a cheap suit, smoking, spitting lyrics at unseen journalists.

Born in 1981 in Detroit, Brown is a true child of the Reagan Revolution. The transformations of Reaganomics were radical, as they were during Thatcherism in the UK and Rogernomics in New Zealand. It was a wholesale embrace of the free-market logic and self-interest espoused by Milton Friedman and his fellow neoliberal economists. A tight group of ideologues, they had been trying, since Barry Goldwater in 1964, to get one of their believers into the White House. In Reagan, they'd finally found their man. Arguably, it is only now—after 9/11, after the Global Financial Crisis, after Trump—that we're starting to understand the full consequences of that revolution.

In January 2017, I saw on Twitter that the great British music critic and philosopher, Mark Fisher, had taken his own life, after a years-long battle with depression, which he'd often written about candidly. Fisher had been a writer I'd known of, but he was never a big figure in my intellectual universe. Other writers I respect were devastated, and social media eulogies flowed. That forced me back into Fisher's work, and specifically, to his most important book: a short text from 2009 called *Capitalist Realism*. Written in the immediate wake of the Global Financial Crisis, Fisher's diagnosis of contemporary capitalism's grip on all of us was as bleak as it was brilliant, summed up by the title of his opening chapter (a line borrowed from Slavoj Žižek and Fredric Jameson): 'It's easier to imagine the end of the world than the end of capitalism'.

Capitalist Realism opens with a superb analysis of the 2006 film *Children of Men*, Alfonso Cuarón's adaptation of P.D. James's dystopian novel in which all women have become sterile and no children have been born for almost two decades. Fisher writes:

> It is evident that the theme of sterility must be read metaphorically, as the displacement of another kind of anxiety. I want to argue this anxiety cries out to be read in cultural terms, and the question the film poses is: how long can a culture persist without the new? What happens if the young are no longer capable of producing surprises?

The central premise of *Children of Men*, Fisher suggests, is that 'that the end has already come'. Such anxieties, he wrote,

> tend to result in a bi-polar oscillation: the 'weak messianic' hope that there must be something new on the way lapses into the morose conviction that nothing new can ever happen. The focus shifts from the Next Big Thing to the last big thing—how long ago did it happen and just how big was it?[3]

There is, I think, a strong correlation between Fisher's analysis of *Children of Men* and Brown's 2016 album *Atrocity Exhibition*. The album is a perfect illustration of capitalist realism in action: a brutal portrait of a black man treading water in contemporary America. Despite his talent and wealth, there's nowhere for Brown to go except deeper into his own depression and anxiety. The album's overriding mood is of a slow panic

---

3   Fisher, 3.

attack: Brown's belief that things should be better than they are, and his inability to cope with the stark fact that no matter how hard he strives for greatness, or for new forms of hip-hop, the world seems not to notice. The world, including his own musical heroes, just sees him as a junked-up, drunk weirdo.

The album's opening track, 'Downward Spiral', is Brown's account of sweating in a room for three days, paranoid, ignoring phone calls, grinding his teeth, hiring prostitutes yet being unable to perform. The song describes pointless financial transactions that promise a happiness and escape that are never delivered. The video that accompanies the song 'Ain't it Funny' is even more confrontational. Directed by the actor Jonah Hill and taking the form of an 80s sitcom, Brown plays the only black character—Uncle Danny. The sitcom's storyline is that Uncle Danny's cries for help for his depression and drug addiction go unheard, much to the hilarity of the all-white studio audience. Towards the end of the video, Uncle Danny, presumably experiencing a horrific trip, is stabbed in the stomach by a giant Xanax pill.

It seems pretty obvious to me that *Atrocity Exhibition* is about the depression and anxiety that are produced not despite neoliberalism's promises of economic freedom and success but because of them. Brown often speaks about his desire to create something that will stand the test of time, something that will bring about the 'shock of the new', and when the culture fails to notice what he's doing, he turns to physical and chemical relief not for pleasure, but for erasure.

One of the most important passages in *Capitalist Realism* deals with a different kind of chemical relief from anxiety's effects: the widespread prescription of Selective Serotonin Reuptake Inhibitors (SSRIs). 'The current ruling ontology,' Fisher wrote, denies any possibility of a social causation of mental illness. The chemico-biologization of mental illness is of course strictly commensurate with its depoliticization. Considering mental illness an individual chemico-biological problem has enormous benefits for capitalism. First, it reinforces Capital's drive towards atomistic individualization (you are sick because of your brain chemistry). Second, it provides an enormously lucrative market in which multinational pharmaceutical companies can peddle their pharmaceuticals (we can cure you with our SSRIs). It goes without saying that all mental illnesses are neurologically *instantiated*, but this says nothing about their *causation*. If it is true, for instance, that depression is constituted by low serotonin levels, what still needs to be explained is why particular individuals have low levels of serotonin. This requires a social and political explanation; and the task of repoliticizing mental illness is an urgent one if the left wants to challenge capitalist realism.[4]

This passage had a double-impact on me when I first read it in early 2017. It helped me understand why I might have ended up on SSRIs, while also convincing me that I needed to get off them as soon as I could.

By that stage, I'd been taking Citalopram—a widely prescribed SSRI in New Zealand—for a few months. My therapist had actually cautioned me against it: we'd been trying variations of CBT tactics for several months. But when they weren't working, my GP decided SSRIs were worth a shot.

The early stages of the treatment were punishing—a days-long and relentless enhancement, rather than diffusion, of pre-existing paranoia. Then there was the shaking: tremors that took over my arms, especially in the mornings. In hindsight, these side effects seemed to support Fisher's argument about the inescapability of capitalism's negative

[4] Fisher, 37.

consequences. At the time, though, they were just terrifying; a failure of body at a moment when, with my enhanced paranoia, I seemed to be suffering from a failure of character, too.

Once my system adjusted to the drug, there was an even wider range of weird effects. The light that caught in the corners of my eyes after a few drinks was brighter and sharper. Smoking marijuana (no, I didn't tell my GP or my therapist) became that little bit better, too; the slow tip-forward of my brain lasting just slightly longer than usual. Sex on Citalopram was like swimming too deep underwater, then feeling your lungs search for the last bit of oxygen as you scramble back to the surface.

Of course, my doctor hadn't told me about these things. And the uncomfortable truth is not all of these effects were terrible. All of it was a damn sight better than my brief experiment with that other family of drugs often prescribed for extreme anxiety: benzodiazepine. The effect of benzos on panic attacks is extraordinary: a near-instantaneous, heroin-like hit that turns your brain to soup. Benzos are, in this sense, glorious. And for that reason, I realised, they are also to be avoided at all costs, especially for anyone with the remotest predisposition to addiction.

For me, SSRIs made some things worse, but they made a lot of things better, and some of those things square up with Brown's approach to sex and intoxication. I wondered about the possibility that it wasn't the Citalopram itself, but its consequences, that were enabling the positive effects I was feeling: that all the drug was doing for me was recalibrating the serotonin in my brain. In effect, was I simply experiencing the kind of present-ness and peace that the majority of the population already experienced day to day? And, Lord, weren't they all lucky if that was the case?

The conundrum I was left with, after reading Fisher's critique of Big Pharma's exploitation of our inability to cope with the world, was this: if we really can't imagine the end of capitalism, and capitalism is what causes mental illness, what are we supposed to do? Why not just take the drugs and escape, even if it only makes us happy for a little while?

This, I began to recognise, was the truth at the heart of Brown's music, which I had found myself listening to more than anything else during this time. The city Brown grew up in—one I've spent a lot of time in and love dearly—plays an essential part in this too, embodying the realities of capitalist realism to a degree few American cities approach: Detroit. The victory of Friedman's revolution was to transform America from a Fordist economy, in which workers, unions and industrialists entered into a kind of co-dependent arrangement—giving the working classes some power and the ability to make a 'living', at least—to a post-Fordist one of outsourcing and job insecurity. This was sold to the masses as free choice, flexibility and meritocracy. Work hard, and you too can be rich. Why be held back by your neighbours, by taxes, by your coworkers and your employer? This was flagrant bullshit that made a handful of people extraordinarily wealthy and left most others flailing. Detroit today is a literal embodiment of that process: the city where Fordism was born and where its subsequent decline scarred it so deeply that it has fallen from one of America's richest cities to one of its poorest: a late-capitalist ruin.

Some commentators have suggested that, given the regular and extreme references to drug use in his music, Brown's use of Reagan and Bush footage points to their failed 'war on drugs'. Their attempts to crack down on the narcotics trade just made the problems worse, particularly for African-American communities. As jobs disappeared, addiction rates went up, especially to pernicious substances like crack cocaine and methamphetamine. It's hard not to see Brown waving a finger at the Reagan–Bush administrations for this. But he is also, I think, pointing to the larger 'success' of those administrations:

that, despite the depth of destruction to working-class cities and communities and to people of colour, they created a society where, as Fisher pointed out, people can't imagine a world without the economic system they created—the very one that keeps us all in chains.

The solution that Brown offers on *Atrocity Exhibition* is a managed intake of chemicals. Obliterating your ego, he seems to say, at least provides temporary relief from the pervasive cruelties of capitalism. Granted, this isn't ideal, or even idealistic. The irony is that this escape is precisely where Brown has found new form: his 'shock of the new' comes when he tells us so starkly that we are all strung up by a system we've agreed to; that we're all just treading water. And, perhaps, this is an implicit call to action. The poisons Brown puts into his body re-emerge as a cultural antidote: to the relentless demands that we be happy with our lot, that we find personal motivation and growth and progress everywhere we look, and that we pretend the world isn't completely fucked up. It's reassuring to hear in his lyrics that you can sink under the rubble and the ruins for a while. It might not cheer you up, but it might make you feel better.

In memory of Mark Fisher, 1968–2017

Fake It Till You Make It

Eamonn Marra

Comedy typically requires a certain amount of bravado—understandable given the immediate and terrifying nature of performing. Eamonn Marra appeared to have no bravado at all.
—Brannavan Gnanalingam, *Lumiere Reader*[1]

A few years ago a girl told me that I had to be more confident, because girls think that confidence is sexy, and that I should fake it till I make it. But I don't want to have to fake something for a girl to find me sexy. I want a girl who thinks that I'm sexy for me, I want to find a girl who thinks that panic attacks are really sexy. Also what does 'fake it till you make it' mean? My anxiety manifests itself in very physical ways; I shake a lot and I sweat a lot, and I don't know how to fake being dry. Also, I'm not sure if I want to stop shaking because it's currently about 80% of the exercise I get.

That is a piece of stand-up comedy from my 2014 New Zealand International Comedy Festival show *Man on the Verge of a Nervous Breakdown*, a show about anxiety performed by someone with great anxiety, without trying to hide it. 'Fake it till you make it' has not worked for me when it comes to anxiety, because I am not a good actor. It left me upset, exhausted and more anxious. It was only when I accepted and acknowledged my anxiety that I managed to get a hold of it enough to move forward with my life, and that came through

[1] 'A Comedy Festival Dispatch: James Nokise, Eamonn Marra, Alexander Sparrow, Tighty Whiteys, Kraken, Juan, two?', *Lumiere Reader*, 12 May 2014. lumiere.net.nz/index.php/j-nokise-e-marra-a-sparrow-tighty-whiteys-kraken-juan-two/

performing stand-up comedy.

I started performing stand-up in 2012, when I was 22 years old. I had just made a life-changing move from my hometown, Christchurch, which had been shaking near constantly for over a year, to a house with precarious foundations on Mount Victoria in Wellington that shook every time a gust of wind hit it.

In post-quake Christchurch—2011, after years of ups and downs, my anxiety had spiralled out of control. I was equally afraid of leaving the house and being home alone, so would push myself out to parties, faking it till I would get a panic attack, drink my way through it, and return home so exhausted I wouldn't be able to leave the house for five days.

The earthquakes in Christchurch had shown me how insignificant people were in the scheme of things, but also their resilience and importance of community. I took part in the Student Volunteer Army but I couldn't deal with the crowds of people and the ongoing and constant reminders of what had happened, so I stopped. I dropped out of two of the three classes I was taking at university and reapplied for WINZ and stopped leaving the house, feeling so guilty that I couldn't do more to help. Every time I was left alone with my thoughts, the same conversation would play out in my head:

Q. 'What am I doing to make this world a better place?'
A. 'Nothing.'
Q. 'What am I doing to make the world a worse place?'
A. 'Quite a lot.'
Q. 'What am I doing to minimise my negative effects on the world?'
A. 'Not enough.'

Then I would make a pact with myself to go vegan, or to shop only at small locally owned stores, or to give $20 of my benefit money every week to charity, or to somehow stop using fossil fuels, but it would never be enough. My existence was causing harm to the world, and there were no changes I could make to make up for it. So every day I would wake up and slowly make the world a worse place. The only solution, I thought, was that it would be better for me to be dead than alive.

After I told this to my counsellor, I spent some time in a mental health respite centre (which later became the basis of a comedy show, *Respite*) and I was put on a high dose of a drug called Quetiapine, which I was instructed to take when I got too anxious. Every time I had these thoughts I would take one of these pills, which were also a sedative, and I would zombie out. So I spent a good eight months living life as a zombie.

Sometime during that eight months, I decided to move to Wellington. Almost as soon as I moved I started doing stand-up. People have asked me why I started and I don't really know. When I came off that dose of Quetiapine in mid 2012, I was a comedian.

Around the same time I started doing stand-up comedy, I also started doing mindfulness therapy. While I never quite committed to listening to those mp3s of Eckhart Tolle telling me to relax (much to my counsellor's dismay), I did take a lot of the points of mindfulness to heart. I learned to pay attention and to acknowledge my feelings as they arose, but I did not let them dictate my actions.

This was quite a big change from my previous strategy of trying to ignore the feelings. That acknowledgement of my anxiety was the biggest step towards being able to manage it.

When I started doing stand-up comedy, it was immediately obvious that the false bravado that many newbies use was never going to work for me. My anxiety was so uncontrollable and all-encompassing that I would have been given away instantly. So instead I used my anxiety in my comedy. I made jokes about panic attacks and social awkwardness. I had routines about how difficult WINZ meetings were and how I struggled to leave the house. I delivered my jokes while reading from a piece of paper, shaking uncontrollably, staring straight at the ground.

The best option was to acknowledge my anxiety. To take a moment to feel it, understand my body's reaction to it, then continue on doing what I want to do. By acknowledging and responding to my feelings of anxiety live in the moment, it not only enabled me to perform comedy in the first place, it made me a better comedian. Those skills of paying attention to your surroundings and a crowd, and adapting are essential for crafting good stand-up, and they're incredibly hard to learn.

I now teach stand-up comedy, and I tell my students to use their unique positions to their advantage. If a comedian talks about their own experiences in a way that is honest to those experiences, they will inherently be engaging and watchable. A comedian who is comfortable onstage is going to be far less funny talking about their panic attacks than someone who can't make eye contact. My honest portrayal of anxiety became my point of difference.

Comedy was a way for me to take control of my life back from anxiety. Anxiety had nearly caused me to drop out of university, it left me unable to work, unable to leave the house or form relationships. Comedy let me prove to myself, and the rest of the world that it hadn't beaten me.

I have often been asked if my onstage anxiety is an act. A lot of people cannot comprehend why someone with anxiety would go out of their way to do something that would cause great anxiety. But as an anxious person with elements of agoraphobia, I have gotten good at doing things that make me anxious. Just leaving the house can push me up to a six or seven out of ten. Running late for something puts me at an eight. It's not too hard to go from that to a nine or ten when I'm performing; whereas for someone who isn't anxious all the time, the jump from a reasonably comfortable two or three to an eight is unfathomable. Even if they're less anxious than me onstage, they're not used to it. They don't know how to cope.

The jokes I wrote in my first few years in stand-up became

the basis of my first one-hour show, *Man on the Verge of a Nervous Breakdown*, which was an entirely accurate title. My first review stated, 'He was lucky there were no hecklers in the room—that would have completely thrown him. He managed to do that all by himself.'[2]

I spent years trying to fake not being anxious, and that just caused more problems. So I prefer be anxious and do it anyway. It wasn't always successful, but I got through it. In comedy failure is inevitable; the best comedians out there still bomb sometimes.

After the initial failure and negative review for the first night of *Man on the Verge of a Nervous Breakdown*, I learned from it and kept going. By the end of the season, the show had transformed. In his review Brannavan Gnanalingam wrote, 'This brilliant show managed to turn depression, loneliness, and anxiety into something that was at once funny and sad, rich and deeply moving.' I managed to turn a failure into something people really engaged with and I couldn't have done without experiencing what it was like to fail first.

People's responses to my comedy about anxiety were heartwarming. Every time someone who had anxiety told me my comedy was important to them it made me feel like I was doing something to make a positive change in the world.

Once my anxiety became more manageable, I became worried that I was losing my point of difference. Could I continue to tell my jokes about anxiety when it was no longer a major part of my day to day life? The jokes no longer hit as hard as they once did; they were less believable. I found myself purposefully playing it up onstage, or inducing anxiety by drinking large amounts of caffeine shortly before I got onstage. I felt like a fraud. I was faking it, but I wasn't sure I had anything to say that wasn't about anxiety.

---

2   Tim Gruar, *Groove Guide*, May 2014.

For the 2018 New Zealand International Comedy Festival, I debuted a new show, *Dignity*. *Dignity* was about what happens after mental illness. I wanted to prove to myself and others that I could do a show that didn't use vulnerability as a crutch, that was just jokes about the world I live in. I wrote an hour of comedy about jobs, fast-food restaurants and money. It was still personal, but it was joyous and fun and looked out at the world rather than inwards. I used the skills I had crafted making jokes about my anxiety and it felt great.

Then between the Auckland season and the Wellington season of *Dignity* I had a breakdown. I was faced with the challenge of performing a show I had written and first performed when I was feeling really good, while I was feeling really bad. I had to fake it. I had to bring an energy to the stage that I did not feel offstage. In the days leading up to the show, I was dreading it. I was trying to maintain a face of enthusiasm to sell tickets but fearing that I couldn't possibly keep that up for an hour onstage. In the final days of rehearsal, I realised I didn't have to. I could write it into the show, and let people know that I wasn't feeling great about it. It not only made it possible for me to perform the show—it made it a lot better.

It Needs to Start Early

An Interview with Riki Gooch

In April 2018 I sat down with Riki Gooch to talk about his experiences with anxiety. I first met Rik back in 2002 through my husband David, who is also a musician. Rik is a phenomenal performer and composer, and he is the funniest, most quick-witted person I know. Over the years I have seen a dark side of him, which comes from the pain of his early childhood trauma. In the past three years he's become open and honest about his state of mind and about his own failures. I wanted to talk to Rik about anxiety because I think he has a lot to offer through his experiences and learning. His story is a tough one, but his resilience and determination to grow and heal himself are insightful, and I hope his words will be encouraging to people who are struggling with trauma and anxiety.
—Kirsten McDougall

KM: What would you say to people who don't have this condition or don't understand it? How could you help them to understand what it's like?
RG: I wonder how many people live without anxiety? It can't be that many! So, to the one person out there without anxiety who is reading this . . . Stuff you! [*laughs*]

The best way to understand what anxiety is to imagine your biggest fear, whether that's standing in front of your classroom and realising you've got no pants on, or being chased upstairs by someone and you can't get away . . . Now imagine putting that under a microscope. While you're looking at it through the lens, it jumps out of the microscope, straight onto your face and suffocates you so you can't breathe, and you can't pull it off—that's anxiety, that's what it feels like.

Do you know what causes your anxiety?
The root of my anxiety comes from early childhood development and sits under the umbrella of post-traumatic stress disorder (PTSD). This stems from abuse I suffered as a child: sexual, physical and emotional abuse. The thing with PTSD is it can cause you to make bad decisions and act in ways that increase anxiety. This might be a behaviour that happens within a relationship or, say, I might make a decision where I buy something to feel better, but then I've just spent the money that was for the kids and then I get anxious.

When did you first start to experience anxiety?
When I was 10 or 11 years old, I felt myself getting really withdrawn. I was just coming out of an abusive childhood and trying to find my way in the world, but I wasn't feeling like I fitted in anywhere. I couldn't make sense of anything. Thankfully, I think anxiety pushed me into the world of music and that's where I've found a calming place, where I feel grounded.

Growing up in Dunedin, as beautiful as it is, the neighbourhood of Corstorphine was pretty shit. There was a lot of gangs around and it was rough. I wasn't a tough kid at all, so every time I stepped out of the house I felt anxious. I had some friends I'd play with every now and then, but music was the only thing that helped. I didn't really notice I had anxiety until I got older. Back then, all I knew was that I would become really withdrawn and I had trouble communicating. My brain was trying to play catch-up.

What did you think was happening to you at the time?
I don't know. I just knew something wasn't right. I knew I was

different, especially in high school, where everybody seemed normal and stable but me. I felt like an outsider and that created anxiety in me.

The crazy thing about anxiety is that it's a loop that goes round and round, so you get anxiety about having anxiety. As a teenager, especially, when you're developing hormonally and are in that transition period to becoming an adult—it was just a nightmare. During that time the anxiety was really building and I was working hard on my music, dedicating myself. But anxiety was also steering me into the dark side of the music scene, which was alcohol and drugs. Even when I was at school, I found comfort in those things. I guess that's where my abuse of drugs and alcohol started.

I started meeting other musicians who had the same bad behaviours as me and who I suspect now also experienced anxiety. I think these people attract each other. There's some weird magnetism that happens between people with early onset of mental-health problems. The drugs and alcohol were self-medication, although at the time I took them under the guise of being cool. Whatever it was, it just worked at the time. When you're 17 years old you have no concept of what might happen to your brain by the time you're 40. You just want to get as fucked up as you can, because all of a sudden it's like, you're cool and you don't feel anxious anymore.

Can you describe a time when your anxiety stopped you from doing something that you wanted to do or needed to be doing?
There's been hundreds of times I've blown opportunities in regards to work. I've had some really good opportunities as a musician, but because I couldn't take care of my mental hygiene, I fucked it. I'd go back to the self-medicating ritual and turn to drugs and alcohol to ease anxiety. Alcohol and drugs make my condition worse, flaming up my bipolar disorder and PTSD and lowering the threshold of my behaviour.

I guess it's now, at the age of 42, that I'm starting to get a concept of what anxiety is and that it's okay. You have to learn to dance with the anxiety instead of trying to drum it out.

Have you been able to talk friends and whānau about your anxiety?
It's been crucial for me to talk about my mental health, but it wasn't always the case that I could. When my daughter was born, 12 years ago, that's when things started to come to a crunch because, when you have a baby, you can't just be some floundering idiot, wreaking havoc everywhere. There's this pressure to be onto it. When my daughter turned up, it opened this can of worms, in terms of my own childhood. My own fears about safety were now projected onto her. I'd worry—who's going to protect her? What am I going to do? This caused anxiety and things really started to spiral out of control.

Over the past ten years I've tried to talk to people about it, but it's only been in the past few years—when my behaviour has had quite dire consequences in terms of the law—that I've had to address anxiety and talk to friends for support. If I can see myself getting stressed, a part of my wellness plan is to talk to my friends and to let them know how I'm feeling.

I think one of the biggest enemies to any mental illness is not talking to friends. Talking takes the sting out of it because all of a sudden your worries become external. I'm really grateful I've got such beautiful friends who will listen; I'm very lucky.

Has the way you experience anxiety changed over time?
Yeah, it has. In the past, it wreaked havoc on my life—like, me being the super drunk guy at an event and being annoying, not paying bills, being useless in relationships. Somehow I maintained a career—I don't know how. I was really self-centred and I struggled a lot. I was a lost soul.

I guess it's really only being over the past few years I've felt this huge transformation in myself. This was forced by events that were serious in my life, life-and-death kinds of situations. At one point, I felt like I was pushed right down to the verge of being suicidal. I wanted to step off. I'd never actually felt that feeling before and I didn't understand how powerful it can be. That's anxiety at its ugliest and most powerful—that saturation of thought and feeling, like you're being bombarded and you can't come up for air. I'm on the other side of that now. The journey my life has taken—it's a blessing. All the stuff that happened shaped me into a better human being.

What kinds of things help ease your anxiety?
Learning what caused my anxiety and PTSD was important. I needed to look back to my difficult childhood, to confront it in order to live with it and make it workable.

Every week I see a clinical psychologist and I do a treatment called EMDR (eye movement desensitisation rehabilitation). This reworks the limbic system in the brain to help deal with traumatic events and responses. It's debated in psychology whether it really works, but I've found it helpful.

I also do CBT (cognitive behavioural therapy), which helps deal with childhood experiences of trauma. Trauma can trigger anxiety; after a traumatic event, your brain gets programmed into reacting a certain way. Even if the trauma happened when you were a child and you're now an adult, the brain doesn't differentiate—it just does its thing. For example, say something bad happened to you when you were little and Dire Straits was playing on the radio. Even 40 years later, when you hear Dire Straits it can trigger an emotion which then creates a behaviour and a consequence—the cycle goes round and round. So CBT is learning about triggers and stopping anxiety before it spirals out of control.

The other thing that's helped my anxiety is going to a drug and alcohol counsellor every week. I've been sober and free from any drugs for over a year now and that's been huge. It's been really hard. Last time I was touring, I had major anxiety attacks, but I didn't go to the usual coping mechanisms of drinking and drugs, and it made me realise how much I was living with these anxiety attacks. I had to ride them out sober and it was awful, but I feel strong now that I'm free from all that stuff.

I have a wellness plan. I've got to make sure my medication is right, make sure that I'm getting enough sleep, make sure I'm eating well and exercising, staying sober. The wellness plan is so essential for me. Everybody can have a wellness plan—you can make your own. If you know you get bad anxiety, you could write down reminders to be gentle on yourself, write up the things that give you comfort when you're feeling bad, like changing your diet, going for a walk, being near water; whatever it is, write it down and put it where you'll see it regularly.

Talking helps, too. With all these things together, staying on top of your health can be a full-time job.

The biggest thing I've been doing lately is meditation and chanting. That's helped me be present and feel fulfilled. It helps me not to feel stuck in the past and badly affected by it, or anxious about the future.

Meditation and chanting helps me know that I am here, in the room with my feet on the ground. I sit and breathe and listen. I remember that I am this mass of flesh and meat and bone, and I'm taking up only a bit of space and hopefully doing some good shit in the world.

Can you describe your experiences with doctors and therapists?
I've been really lucky with therapists. I know that the mental health system in New Zealand is struggling. I'm so grateful for every bit of help my therapists give me each week, because I know there are people in worse condition than me.

It's been a different story with some of the doctors and psychiatrists. They definitely come from more of a medical angle—it's all about medication and it's very clinical. They're analysing and looking at your brain chemistry and trying to work out what's happening. They'll see you as having a chemical imbalance and will compose a chemical cocktail so you can plonk out. That has its benefits—I'm definitely not talking that down—but I think you also need a holistic approach—whether it's a yogi, psychologist, CBT therapist or a priest. Likewise, if you're just going to a psychologist, you may need to see a doctor as well, to find out what's going on chemically in your brain. I do think it's important to be proactive and to explore as many things as possible in order to have a balance between the clinical world and what you might call the spiritual world.

I'm interested in where your experience with treatment, which has been quite positive, intersects with the fact that you are Māori. Stats say that Māori adults are about 1.5 times as likely as non-Māori adults to report a high or very high probability of having an anxiety or depressive disorder, with Māori males twice as likely as non-Māori males to report it. How did you get to the point where you could ask the help? What's the difference between you and the Māori men in these stats?

I definitely live a more privileged life than a lot of other Māori men. Just thinking about the Māori men and women in my family who have suffered horrible mental illness, there's a high rate of suicide which goes back generations. I think I'm different because the world of music opened up networks of opportunities and people for me. I feel that I am more Pākehā in my ways than I am Māori. If I go back and see the family, I feel like the whitest guy there. When I was growing up I felt like I was too brown for the white kids and too white for the brown kids, and this was a cause of anxiety.

Now, I guess it's almost a class thing that I've had more opportunities. Through music, I've had the privilege of access to networks. For example, the doctor and poet Glenn Colquhoun was the first person to recognise there was something wrong with me. We were doing an arts project together, and if not for meeting him and talking to him through that, I wouldn't have spoken to a doctor, and through my doctor I wouldn't have met my psychologist. If I had just been living in South Dunedin, struggling with all this stuff, I'd probably be in prison or hospital or dead. When I say I've been privileged, I don't mean that I live like a privileged person but that I feel privileged because I've had these opportunities through music.

What do you think these statistics say about being Māori?
There is a massive issue with Māori mental health. The Māori mental health unit [Te Whare Marie] is saturated with fellow Māori who are struggling. I think historical trauma has been passed down through DNA, through culture, through colonisation and its effects. With any colonial movement there is huge displacement, not just of land and people, but of identity and spirit. It gets passed down through generations. Māori would call it mākutu, which is a curse that carries on until it is broken. I think there's been a devastating effect on Māori through losing connection with the land and with whakapapa, connection with simplicity and with your spiritual realm, with how you fit in—your tūrangawaewae. Losing those connections means you are walking in between worlds, which translates to mental health issues. Quite often these are spiritual issues.

It is interesting with statistics when they say, If you're a Māori man you're more likely to die at this age, and you'll most likely to end up with a mental health condition or being in jail ... We're doing really well in the statistics—we are winning those! It feels like there's no other way round the devastating effects of colonisation.

In saying that, I think there has been a big shift in New Zealand as a community trying to do something about this. It's not like in Australia, where everything has been swept under the carpet. I actually feel like people here really care, just from the fact that we have these statistics and they're in everybody's faces. The suicide rate is crazy. And I know this happens across all cultures—it's not just Māori; it's also the Pākehā working class.

Here is a big question—how do you think we can change these statistics?
We have to start with the schooling system. We have to replace social studies or physical education with things like mindfulness and yoga and meditation, with learning how to learn and how to express feelings. This goes especially for young males, teenage boys who are struggling with hormones and figuring out where they fit in among all this shit they see on the internet.

Start it at an early age. We need to teach kids how to become critical thinkers, how to have self-care and self-awareness, how to encounter the world being more enlightened and highly tuned. We have to stop saturating them in this capitalist world and education system.

Start in the home, as well. For people who have to work three jobs and can't be there for their own children, it's really tough—society is fucked, that it's like that. It all starts in the home, and it all starts at school, that's things can change. We can't rely on picking up the pieces when kids are older and the damage has been done, saying, 'This kid is completely fucked,' then drugging him up only to put him in a home, then let him out, then find him hanging in a park. This is what happens over and over again.

What if you took the same kid at the age of five and taught him meditation? What if you taught him about being still in his mind? Teach him about the importance of the mind and how powerful it is, how bad things can happen in life but you can build up a resistance to it by looking after yourself. Mindfulness should be an important part of education. Because of the lack of mindfulness, we get mental illness, and mental illness causes bad decision-making.

So that's my answer: it needs to start early. With Māori children, get them back home to their whakapapa. It's not necessarily about learning te reo Māori, but it is about learning about where they come from, where they fit into the world.

What could the health system do to better help people with anxiety?
I think the health system needs financial support, because if something is under-resourced, it is hard for people to get the help they need. I also think there needs to be a more holistic approach to helping people, offering multiple solutions. But the system is how you engage with it too—it's really only one part of the equation; most of the work happens outside of the doctor's rooms. Most of the work is done when you go walking in the trees and when you do your meditation—that's the health system. That's how you need to think about your own 'health system'.

Voices

by Donna McLeod

for Ani

So you want to hear our voices on anxiety.

We are the Nannies, the Aunties, the mothers, the daughters.
We live in our Mana Wāhine,
in Te Ao Mārama and Te Ao Pākehā.
Most of us live in the between.
We uphold the mana of the whenua,
we uphold the mana of the iwi,
we uphold the mana of the whānau.
We uphold that sacred space as Wāhine Māori.
We hold space.

Often while being marginalised by many of our own:
our koro, uncles, fathers, husbands and sons.
We stand and karanga and kīnaki
and we listen time and time again while our men whakamana
each other, darting across the paepae, stroking one another's
importance, reciting words that signify nothing.
You have forgotten what our Nannies taught you
but can conveniently drop their name when needed.
To stand on them and be raised on their shoulders.
But what shoulders Mana Wāhine carry.
We balance you.
We hold space.

And in Te Ao Pākehā you question our Māoriness.
Quantify our Māori blood. Half caste, quarter caste, full?
Qualify our academic qualifications and give us scores out of 10.
We strive to be nice, pretty Māori girls but are often called rude and aggressive.
We hold space.

We smile and calm our taniwha as you practise your te reo Māori on us. Your understanding of Te Tapa Whā, and your best friend or aunty who married a Māori.

We breathe.
We hold space.

We, too, celebrate our Irish, Scottish, French, Spanish tīpuna from the four winds. We celebrate our children travelling the world to send photos of old churchyards, where part of us rests too.
Yet our round brown faces aren't always a welcomed cousin in your eyes.
But whakapapa is everything. The only thing.
We stand. We exhale.
In Aotearoa we are born of this whenua; we are born of its people. We are Māori.
The kaitiaki of people and lands.
We stand.

So how goes your maunga,
your awa,
your whenua,
your standing place,
your people?
And how is it that when I am the only Māori woman in a room, I need to have expertise on resource consent, on your uncle

who found a waka on his farm, on 1080, on the Moriori, on water consent, on the scholarships Māori get, on your great-great-grandfather who married a Māori princess?

We stand.
We smile.

Why, when we welcome you into our homes, do you ask if we are renting? *Oh, you own it, for how long? Lucky you, to get a Māori Affairs loan. Gee, you Māoris are lucky.*
We stand.
We offer cake.

Why, when we drive a Rover, a Jaguar or a Lexus, do the police stop us to ask *Do you own this vehicle?*
We hold space.
We hold silence.
Why, when my whanaunga arrive in two cars with their babies and children, do two police cars arrive with six policemen, after receiving a call from a frightened neighbour regarding a gang gathering?
We hold space.
We choose our battles.
Transcripts are sourced.
Police apologies are made.
The neighbour is to remain anonymous.
We hold space.

How do you serve your people?
Your manaaki?
Your awhi?
We leave our warm beds at the ring of a phone, a text, to sit with whānau who need us to hold their mum's hand as she leaves this world.

We pick up the hair on the floor that our moko cut from his head before he hung himself.

We are the voices that keep time as a koro breathes, waiting for his moko to rush across the world and be there.
We hold our boy and girl babies to our chests as they confide in us the secrets that no child should hold.
We are the ones who confront the monsters.
We are the ones who take razor blades and knives from bleeding wrists as our babies struggle with the bodies they are trapped within.
We remove our mokopuna from our children we have lost to P.
We hold space.
We embrace Wāhine Toa.

We arrive first with the toilet paper, tea bags, milk, sugar.
We set up kitchens in sheds, under tarps, in all weathers.
We can serve 200 people at the drop of a hat
if need be taking food from our own children.
Our hands receive koha; our hands are koha; our feet are swollen. We reach for a V, a fag, sugar.
We hold space.
We laugh.
We are rich, we are poor; who knows, who cares.
Fish, pigs, sheep, chicken, kūmara, potatoes, pumpkin.
All an act of faith, a neighbour, a friend, a cousin.
We wheel, we deal, we beg, we borrow.
We make something from nothing.
We stand, we uphold the mana.

We are the ones whose hearts break.
When the headlines are of murder, rape, child abuse
we unite in a prayer: *Don't let the victim nor the perpetrator be one of ours.*

Our oneness as New Zealanders dissipates in the light of our tomorrows.
We must justify ourselves, our culture, our being. We are police show superstars. We have Māori features, we are light-skinned Māori, dark-skinned Māori, part Māori.
In the negative stats, we are Māori.
We must justify our culture, our being, ourselves.
We prepare to give away part of our souls
to stand in our workplaces, schools, communities.
We armour up. *Bloody Māoris. Horis, what do you expect. Only good Māori is a dead one.*
For comic relief we have the Honourable Hone Carter, the Honourable John Banks, a funny Bob Jones article, a Hobsons Pledge petition at your neighbourhood pie shop.

For wāhine Māori, there is no neutral.
We laugh.
Our fight or flight is to stand,
to hold space.

So we stand before you.
Yes, we have anxiety.
Yes, we have panic attacks.
We don't sleep.
But we hold space
and in that space
we await you.

Author's note: *This is my community's voice. In writing this piece, I thought of all the women I have witnessed holding that sacred space. I sent it to other Māori women to read and all found it emotionally difficult, because our voice isn't often heard or seen. They recognised themselves and their Nannies, Aunties and mothers in this piece. Many of these stories are known; we live them.*

Showing Up

Hinemoana Baker

The proper term for what I do is *dermatillomania*. I bite my fingernails, and I also pick at the cuticles and skin around them until they bleed. I've done it since I was a child. I have tried painting them with bitter Stop 'n Grow, putting Band-Aids around my fingertips and wearing gloves, even in the height of summer. Each of these methods works for a short while, but eventually I'm back in the habit. Meeting new people, I'm ashamed to extend my hand for a handshake. I have long fingers and strong, expressive hands, but I rein them in, trying to keep my hands hidden. The insides of my pockets are flecked with spots of blood.

Some people who live with this behavioural symptom of anxiety pick at other parts of their bodies—their faces, limbs or scalps. It's a form of OCD, the doctors say, fuelled by a desire to smooth things out, to fix imperfections. For me it's more of a release—perhaps similar to the feeling people have after other forms of self-harm.

I don't remember anxiety as a child so much as I do depression. I was 14 when I first wanted to kill myself. I chose a day, and after school I walked through the orchard behind my house saying goodbye to the trees and the birds. I was sad and determined.

Lots of things had led to this. My parents split up after a 27-year marriage marked by my father's violence and affairs, and my mother and I moved from Whakatāne to Nelson. Not long after that I was raped by a boy I had a crush on at my new high school. It isn't the only time I've been raped, but it remains a defining moment in my young life. I had never had sex before, so that was how I lost my virginity.

Mum and I lived with an aunt who was not fond of teenagers, and who bullied my mother. I didn't tell anyone about the boy raping me. I felt my mother had enough problems already.

On this chosen day I walked into the sleep-out Mum and I shared at my aunty's house, dumped my bag in my room and went straight for the safety-razors. I stood at the bathroom sink. It was hard to get the blades out of the plastic fittings they were in—for, you know, shaving—so I left them in there and tried my best. I knew I had to slice lengthways, not across, so I would cut the veins and not just the tendons. At least that was the received wisdom among the other teenagers I knew.

I cut, but it felt like it wasn't happening fast enough, and it hurt. I heard Mum walk in the door but I couldn't really do anything; I could only stand there. She walked in to the bathroom and she was shocked, distraught. I had done quite a bit of bleeding. Fortunately, not enough.

Mum cleaned me up. She cleaned up the bathroom. We cried. Later that day, when we were drinking our cups of tea, she asked me why. Her menthol cigarette was burning away in the big blue ashtray. I said, 'I don't know.'

She said, 'Don't tell your aunty.'

I couldn't bring myself to tell anybody what was going on. I had a part-time job in a dairy in Richmond, after school and on weekends. I was serving customers food, reaching inside the big glass cabinet for cream buns and filled rolls to put into paper bags for their lunch, with thick bandages around my both wrists. No one mentioned it.

Somehow, I was still doing well at school. In fact, the worse things were for me emotionally, the better my marks seemed to get. So in my case, one of the most common triggers for intervention was absent.

Mum was trying to keep everything together. She had been planning to leave Dad for a long time, but was afraid he would take her to court to get custody of me. One day Mum said, 'I'm leaving in two weeks. I'm leaving your father. This will be for good. Who do you want to live with?' I chose her.

I felt terribly guilty, like I had betrayed my father. From the moment Mum told Dad we were leaving till the day we left, he didn't speak to either of us. It was terrifying because his silence was almost always a precursor to an explosion of violence. Not until he was pulling away from the kerb at Whakatāne Airport, then driving off down the long country road that leads away from it, did I feel we were finally safe. I stared after his car, feeling the tarmac burn under the soles of my plastic sandals.

In my 20s, still, it isn't the anxiety I remember, but the rage. I was reckless, thinking, 'If no one gives a fuck about me, why should I?' I ruined friendships and put myself in dangerous situations, while somehow maintaining the illusion of a normal, young life. I remember one boyfriend trying to escape my rage fits by driving away from our flat. I threw myself on the bonnet of his car, screaming.

At other times I was having sex with guys I hardly knew in dark, remote places. Older guys, mostly, and once with a couple I didn't know, having told no one where I was. I had a destructive friendship with the father of a friend, which ended with me walking over the high supporting archway of a concrete bridge that goes over the Maitai River to Nelson. It was, again, late and moonlessly dark. He was shaking when I made it down safely. I wasn't.

In my 30s, the anxiety started to take over. It became free-ranging, one day obsessing about money; the next, about being a terrible friend. I have special scripts written by my anxiety for each of these subjects. They tell me all about what kind of a person I am. At times, I become deliriously anxious about the prospect of suffering another episode of severe depression. I am especially fearful of the bad episodes, where I become catatonic, not able to move easily from one position or location to another.

Not being able to get out of bed, or chairs, or up from the floor or out of the car, is very scary for me. It's more than inertia. It's a physical manifestation of being so overcome by thoughts and doubts that I cannot move in any direction. Even when I'm relatively well, I have a constant background fear of chairs and comfortable surfaces.

Depression and anxiety are cruel, because even though you know the exact things that would make you better, it becomes excruciatingly difficult to do them. Physical movement—getting back in my body—is one of my most effective weapons against anxiety, but instead I end up stuck in a chair or in bed, biting into my fingers till they bleed, obsessively refreshing Facebook. Getting to the swimming pool or being able to exercise can be tricky for a lot of people, but for those of us with anxiety and depression it can feel ludicrous, fantastically impossible. In the next five minutes I may be able to move my left leg three inches so the circulation comes back into my completely numb foot. Clearly, at minute six, I'll be up to 50 lengths of freestyle.

Social situations are another thing my anxiety latches on to. People are often surprised to hear this, because I am a performer and a teacher, and I seem very confident doing those and many other things. I tell them I am good at camouflage. It's survival. One of my closest friends often says to me, 'I've known you for nearly 15 years and I still can't tell when you're having a hard time unless you outright say so.'

Another dear friend of mine throws an annual summer party and she invites me every time. Some years I feel strong enough to drive there, park and turn the car key to OFF. Some years I am then able to open the door of the car and walk into the house. 'Just half an hour,' I say to myself, 'just half an hour.' Several times I have simply driven home, hating myself, adding another instrument to the *you're a terrible friend* orchestra playing in my head.

I was in my 30s when I studied for a Master of Arts at the International Institute of Modern Letters at Victoria University of Wellington. It was a privilege to be accepted, and I was thrilled. But it became difficult to distinguish the anxious, unhelpful, trawling through every single syllable for perfectionism-driven improvements from the legitimate work of receiving feedback and redrafting.

God knows how I got through that year. I didn't write nearly enough and I flagellated myself mercilessly about it. I was in a relationship with another anxious and rageful woman who frayed what remaining nerves I had and made me permanently scared. I boxed on. A year later I had enough material for a book, and then another horrifying thing happened: Viggo Mortensen offered to publish it.

It was indeed a *Luxusproblem*, as we say here in Germany—try to stay with me while I moan about this ridiculously fortunate life event. Viggo was based in Wellington for several years while filming *The Lord of the Rings*, and he fell in love with the place. He wanted to give something back to the city. He is a recognised writer, musician and painter, as well as an actor, a big fan of poetry and, it turns out, of Bill Manhire, our professor. Viggo approached Bill and asked if he could organise a poetry fundraiser for scholarships to the Master's programme. We held an evening where he read a selection of his work alongside Tusiata Avia, Cliff Fell, Bill and me.

Viggo has a publishing company in Santa Monica, co-founded with an art curator named Pilar Perez. They were both focussed on finding someone from New Zealand to publish, and I think the whole Māori thing appealed to them as well—Viggo is a political bloke. A good bloke. He seemed anxious, actually, on the night of the reading. In the green room, he dropped his printed poems all over the floor. Onstage, he was hesitant and still nervous.

I found this all strangely comforting.

When he first asked to publish my work, I thought he was joking, this weird Hollywood actor who goes around the world making promises to new poets. Insanely, I kind of ignored his emails. It turned out he was serious, and he and Fergus Barrowman at Victoria University Press cut a deal so they could co-publish my first book.

It was all too much for my wired, anxious, strung-out brains. Who was it that talked about people being more afraid of success than failure? The whole process of interacting with Viggo about the book was excruciating. I mean, he was lovely—attentive, respectful, had great editorial suggestions—while I was often barely able to respond to his emails, sometimes for weeks at a time, all the while silently screaming at myself. I was trying to be all, 'Oh wow this is so cool,' but inside I was like, 'Argh, I am going to fuck this up any minute!'

Fortunately, both Viggo and Fergus didn't let my tardiness and general insanity affect their commitment to publish. The book, *mātuhi | needle*, turned out well. But Pilar, and I'm sure the others involved, must have been pissed off at times. I don't blame them.

I published two further books after that, as well as putting out a couple of albums, and each project was easier on my anxiety levels. This was thanks, in large part, to wise words and kindness from my writing group and my other artist friends. For ten years or so, I managed, through constant attention and the fact that I was teaching it all the time, to stick with the 'Just turn up and write something every day and the book will take care of itself' strategy. I got good at writing through my anxiety, and in spite of it.

Then, in my late 30s, I began what was to be the longest romantic relationship of my life with a fellow musician, Christine. Soon after, I wanted to try for a baby. I'd left it late, and she wasn't too keen. But I hadn't felt well enough, or in love enough, to try earlier, and I didn't want to do it alone.

It turns out I wasn't one of those people destined to get pregnant first pop. Or even the second, or third. Trying to conceive ('TTC' in all the online forums—dear god, the memories) was uniquely aligned with all the worst aspects of my anxiety. I was project-managing the whole shamozzle myself, due mainly to lack of funds and trust for IVF or other clinic-based processes. Therefore I had to keep finicky records of everything about my cycle and my body. I also took on the role of matching up mine and Chris's diaries with the diary of our donor: all of us self-employed (ack), two of us in the arts (ugh) and therefore all under-resourced in almost every way, including time.

The practicalities of conceiving, though, was nothing compared to managing our emotions and relationships. It is a big deal to have a baby with anyone, let alone on purpose, with someone who isn't your partner but wants to help, while your own partner's ambivalence sometimes manifests as almost sabotaging the whole high-stakes process. Emotionally, legally, financially—trying for a baby was a perfect storm of stress, grief and, of course, anxiety.

Nevertheless, I threw myself into it, because micromanagement felt like a way I could control this completely uncontrollable thing. If I took my temperature at exactly the right moment, and spat on a microscope, and examined the position and openness of my cervix every day of my fertile window, and analysed the exact nature of my secretions, and tested my ovulation hormones, and charted my progress, and wrote down my moods and my dreams, and avoided alcohol, and made sure my donor wasn't smoking weed or riding his bike too much, and relaxed and lay down for two hours after inseminating, making sure to rotate like a rotisserie chicken every 20 minutes after having my legs up the wall for an hour, and avoided sugar and coffee, and relaxed and did yoga, and walked on the beach and emptied my mind, and had acupuncture and took tinctures and flower fucking essences, and didn't overthink it, *then* I would get pregnant.

As time passed, each period began to feel like a death. I couldn't think or talk about anything else. My grief compounded and blossomed anew with every month of not getting pregnant.

Then I did. It happened just before my 40th birthday, for which I had planned a kayaking trip around Tasman Bay with Chris and a couple of very good friends. I miscarried into the long-drop at Observation Beach, one of the beautiful and isolated bays of the Abel Tasman National Park. I spent the rest of the trip howling like an animal and ruining everyone's holiday.

I was 43 when I finally gave up on conceiving. My relationship with Chris ended then, after nine years. In the same year, I was chosen as the 2014 Writer in Residence at Victoria University of Wellington. I spent the rest of the residency living in various houses, nothing permanent. I was not writing anything properly because I was so anxious, all the time. I could hardly read, let alone write. But I kept showing up, day after day, feeling sick with nerves and sadness, pretending to be fine.

I was writing another book. This one was about my father, and his abuse at the hands of nuns in Nelson's Sunnybank Orphanage, and also about my infertility. For the Sunnybank side of things, I did some research and came back to Nelson, but right from the beginning the book began to feel terrifying. Its implications began to overwhelm me, and I felt incapable of acquitting myself properly. I wrote about 40,000 words, but none of it felt like it was working, and then I thought, 'Well I will just keep writing this draft and then I'll re-draft it, like proper writers do, after that.' I ran a crowd-funding campaign and people gave me money to do just that. Bless those folks.

When I arrived in Berlin for the 2016 Creative New Zealand Berlin Writers' Residency, fresh from another breakup and dealing with a family illness, I was a bit of a wreck. I travelled via India to see a friend and, in the airport at Bangalore while waiting for my flight to Germany, I had my first major migraine episode. I collapsed in the toilets and had to be revived at the airport's medical clinic. After a couple of hours on a drip of anti-nausea and pain meds, I wobbled off the table. When I got to Berlin, the sickness stayed. I was there on a writing residency, but just looking at a screen brought on overwhelming nausea, my head swimming with pain.

Physical pain has been a part of my anxiety since my 20s. I believe it is somatised anxiety. I also have fibromyalgia, and for many years I required special equipment to be able to type at a desk—arm supports and stuff. These days the fibro is far quieter, kept at bay with weight-training and swimming, but the migraines still mess with me. This essay is the longest single thing I've written in two years.

Nowadays I know enough about my anxiety, its symptoms and effects on my daily functioning, to manage it. I know it flares in a crisis—my mum died a few months ago, which has sent things into overdrive. But I feel a thread of stability returning. And I can start to write again, finish the book I started back in 2014, with its dark, difficult subject matter. It may take more like ten years than two, but that's okay.

Today, it's Friday. It's summer, and I am sitting in the beautiful Staatsbibliothek in Berlin, the old East German State Library. It's a stunning place—as my friend William said, 'It's like walking into the East German Royal Albert Hall.' Outside, it's 31 degrees, and inside it's a perfect 24. I have been here all day working on this essay, and I have had no heart palpitations. I have managed to eat normally, with little nausea. My right index finger is showing signs of my attack on it earlier today, but it's stopped bleeding, and my other fingers are not too shredded.

My shoulders are very tight, as is my neck, and the three smallest fingers on both of my hands are totally numb. The self-hatred tape-loop is running—*No one will ever want to read this, why don't you try putting some happiness into the world instead*—but its volume is lower than usual today, so I have been able to type. I am remembering to breathe, remembering to move regularly—not to be paralysed, not to be scared of my chair. I'm grateful for days like this.

Soon I will leave the library and bike to the nearby gym: a strangely homey, bad-smelling place above a pizza joint at Rosenthaler Platz, where the machines and the carpet tiles have seen better days and so have most of the members, myself included. I will do some exercise, listening to a podcast called 'Griefcast', and I will feel accompanied and understood. Later, I will eat dinner on the banks of the river Spree with a good friend. We will walk beside the water.

Naming

Bonnie Etherington

I learned how to swim underwater before I learned how to swim at the surface. As a child, I regularly dived into the deep end of the community pool and sank on purpose to the bottom, learning how to control the release of my breath, slowing my heartbeat down. I imagined my brainwaves unwrinkling as I did this. Sounds seemed far away. My muscles relaxed and were calm, my jaw unclenched. I was safe in my own world. Other fears—other people—no longer seemed as important. But, always, I had to return to the surface and return to those fears.

My best friend died when I was five. His name was Boni, which is a homonym of my own name, Bonnie. In fiction that would be implausible. Almost every day, I remind myself that he died and I didn't. He was male; I am female. He was Papuan; I am originally from New Zealand. He was only a little older than I was when he died from malaria. I have had malaria many times, as well as other childhood illnesses with consequences that have lasted into adulthood. But I am alive because I was privileged enough to have a nurse for a mother and access to medication. I carry all this information around with me.

I understood that Boni was in the small plywood coffin in front of us at the funeral. In West Papua—called Irian Jaya at the time—death was and still is something you cannot hide from. Boni's family killed a pig for his funeral feast. While it was cooking, some other friends and I blew up the pig's bladder and played with it like it was a balloon. I understood where the bladder came from. I understood that my friend was no longer there to play with. Still, I played. I don't think I cried.

When I first went to see a counsellor I thought I had to figure out which *one thing* in my life had caused me to be the way I am. A part of me thought that Boni's death might be top of the list. I wanted to identify one thing that explained why I have what my mum calls a 'hummingbird heart', why I can't wear headphones outside in case someone comes up behind me, why I have an exit plan for any room I happen to be in, why sometimes I do not leave my apartment for weeks at a time. Why the nightmares, why the excruciating migraines that make me wilt, why I have never, even as a child, been able to sleep well. You've just always been a bit anxious—a worrier, so alert, says my mum. But being 'a bit anxious' has taken many forms.

As a teenager, my anxiety manifested as an eating disorder. I remember one night after showering, at the height of my illness, I caught a glimpse of my back in the mirror. All bones, my body did not feel or look like it belonged to me. The sensation wasn't new: as a child, sometimes I believed I was floating above my body. I would look down and see the top of my head, the rims of my glasses. It was a way to see the things that happened to me but not feel them. Later, when I used the eating disorder to escape my body, I imagined myself shrinking into smaller and smaller spaces. A suitcase, an empty tin, a postage stamp. I could feel safe for a time, like I did in the pool, though again, the feeling never lasted.

Ever since then, I have been learning to fit back in my body, fleshing out each corner. This can be a painful thing. Part of learning to live with the hummingbird heart is in naming what separates me from my body like this, what makes me shrink. There's the anxiety, which has always been with me—a gene passed down a long line of women who have all managed it in their different ways. And then there is this thing called 'complex post-traumatic stress disorder' which grew out of all that. It is not the best of names, but what it describes is PTSD caused by a long-term build-up of things, like snow rising before an avalanche. Over time I concluded there was no *one thing*; it was not Boni. He was not even the beginning.

I do wonder if naming—identifying or diagnosing what and how I feel, using labels such as 'anxiety' and 'PTSD'— is *always* helpful. Are the names just another way to shrink me down and distance myself from my own body and brain? I do not know the whole answer, but I do know there are days when a diagnosis offers me room to understand myself and other days it does not. At the moment, I live in the United States, and too often the evening news blares with the sounds and images of mass shootings. The conversation inevitably turns to mental illness: did the shooter have depression, anxiety, PTSD—you name it. If the answer is yes, everyone has a place to lay the blame. This, I think, is harmful use of the medical terms so many of us live with our whole lives.

It is also important, especially for PTSD (which, for me, is general anxiety's close relative), to know that this label is not only for one kind of person who has had one kind of experience. These disorders can be strange and often amorphous things. Perhaps another answer to the question of naming's worth is that if more of us who live with these disorders as our companions start to name them, then perhaps others will see the expanse of our experiences and we can breathe more easily within these zones of our lives, too—with our knowledge of our dead, our hurts, our many terrors.

Some people have told me I write and think about death too much. They're probably right: the maxim is to write what you know, and I know death. I did my first years of primary school via correspondence, and every day we had to write a story or journal entry. A couple of years ago, I came across these old stories when I was deep in revisions for my first novel—a novel that includes a fairly high death-count because it is set in West Papua and, as I mentioned earlier, to live in West Papua is to be close to death. To be clear, it is also so much more. I am always trying to balance death with life in my writing, but maybe not succeeding. One of the stories I'd written for school was of a man who went to check a pig trap in the forest. He found a pig in the trap, but it had been there for a few days and was very hungry and angry. The man shot it once with an arrow but the pig, instead of dying, broke free. It killed the man and ate part of him. Later, the man's relatives came and killed the pig. They then ate the pig.

This was a true story. I was about seven when it happened. My correspondence teacher did not know how to respond, and she placed a 'Wow!' sticker on the page and mailed it back to me. I find this funny now, but I also put a similar scene in my novel so that I did not feel so alone with this experience. Writing such scenes feels like another way of naming, of asking people to witness and sit with me, just for a short time.

At a literal level, writing makes space for the names of those whom death took. If I do not write about them, then their names come out in other ways, like to an Uber driver or a hairdresser. Even if the hairdresser is nice about it, I'm probably not paying her enough to hear the names of dead people.

But naming can't solve everything. I habitually shower at night but recently, when my husband started working late shifts, I found myself barely able to use the bathroom or the shower when alone in the apartment at night. I was sure that the falling water would mask the sounds of an intruder sneaking up behind me. These were some of my lowest months with anxiety. One day, my husband and I decided to adopt a pet from the animal shelter. A calico cat with wounded back legs, notched ears and half a tail stood out to us. Then we noticed the name on her cage: Bonnee. I laughed.

This one, said my husband. She's the one.

I was doubtful she was the one. The name seemed like too much of a coincidence—and not a good one. When we brought her home it was clear that she had anxiety issues of her own, resulting in puddles of piss every time she was scared, hiding at every sound. We renamed her and set about loving her as best we could. A few months later, I realised I could shower at night again, even if no one else was home. This was a victory. Just the cat's presence and breathing in the same room as mine made the shadows less hostile, the sounds less loud. The cat changed, too. She learned to talk to squirrels outside the window and she likes wedging herself in between my computer and me. The puddles of piss gradually stopped.

Several years ago, I tried scuba diving while in Indonesia. Predictably, before I tipped into the water, I shook and my heart rate was high. But, once submerged, again I felt the sensations that had drawn me to the deep end of the community pool when I was younger. Perhaps it is the pressure of the water or the controlled regular breathing—in and out, never holding air for long—which keeps anxious thoughts from intruding that far underwater. On that first dive, right as I passed over a crowd of angelfish, my equipment malfunctioned at the same time as I inhaled my next breath. My lungs filled with seawater and pain. I remember looking up, seeing how far away the surface of the water was, thinking I would not make it up in time and feeling strangely at peace with this. Without the sound of my breathing I could hear the crackling of parrotfish, the hum of boats somewhere above, the bump of unseen bodies and objects. Around me, the angelfish clustered close, as if they knew. As I started to pass out, lungs still filled with water, our instructor appeared and was able to get a spare air source to me. Later, recovered at the surface, the instructor said she had never seen anyone so calm in a near-death situation. I do not know why then, of all times, I did not panic like my body seems primed to do. Perhaps it was the press of the fish bodies, like my cat presses against me now, easing the anxiety brought on by things I could not name.

There are no tidy endings when it comes to living with anxiety, but there is comfort in other bodies willing you to share their breath and life. There are some things that can be named, in amongst all the things that cannot. There are ways not to feel alone. The bottom of the pool and the bottom of the ocean are just the places that first gave me the space to discover these things.

My husband, my cat, and I—we jokingly call ourselves the PTSD family. We're learning to live with it. Together, we work to name and to fit ourselves back inside our bodies. For me, it feels like being underwater but looking up.

Mrs Housewife

Holly Walker

'Friction stay windows in the living room bring in plenty of sun, while from the kitchen sink Mrs Housewife keeps up with affairs in the neighbourhood,' announces the plummy narrator of a 1954 government newsreel about life in newly built state housing suburbs. 'Here's a space-saver!' he chirps. 'A drop-table hides the stools—an ideal breakfast table for two.' Cheerful strings keep three-four time under the voiceover. Mrs Housewife looks like death warmed up.

My maternal grandmother, Lucy, was a Mrs Housewife too. Until she married (late for those days, in her mid 30s) she led an independent life, full of tennis parties at the family home, trips to the pictures, female friendships and good-natured banter with the blokes at work. One of seven children, she seemed to have accepted that she would be the daughter to remain single and stay at home to help their mother. She liked to have fun, though, so at weekends she would go out dancing. One night at the Majestic Cabaret she met my grandfather, Graham, a widowed travelling salesman with a four-year-old daughter. They won the Monte Carlo together. Almost reluctantly, she was charmed. While she enjoyed her freedom as a single working woman, perhaps she also found the idea of starting a family of her own appealing. They married in 1952.

After only a two-week honeymoon, Graham contracted tuberculosis and was hospitalised. Lucy entered a strange limbo, moving back with her mother for two years as if nothing had changed, only seeing her new husband on visits to the hospital. When he was finally discharged in 1954, the couple were allocated a small state house in the suburban promised land of Naenae, and a different life commenced for Lucy. Thrown into stepmotherhood, she quickly gave birth to two more daughters of her own. Now she was the primary carer for three children, including two under two, in a house that was barely large enough to contain them. She also had to care for Graham, who, in addition to recovering from TB, had type 1 diabetes, Parkinson's disease, ulcerative colitis and two forms of arthritis. She was often required to resuscitate him from one of his diabetic 'turns' to prevent him from requiring hospitalisation. Her new life in the suburbs, as wife of an ailing husband and mother of young children, could not have been more different from that which she had enjoyed just a few years earlier. While she loved her husband and children, it can't have been a smooth transition.

'You get bored when you stay home with the children,' says another Mrs Housewife in a later, less chirpy archival clip. She's feeding a plump baby from a bottle. 'You long for a bit of stimulation, not only with other women but with men, and people in the working community. You somehow get this idea that people who work have a much more interesting life, because they've got other people to talk to . . .'

In Lucy's time, they had a term for the psychological distress that the changes of motherhood often brought: suburban neurosis. Many women self-medicated with alcohol ('mother's little helper'). An official diagnosis might have produced a Valium prescription. Either way, the women of Lucy's generation who were thrown into neurosis by motherhood were encouraged to take the edge off, rather than consider or address the underlying causes of their distress.

For many years I did not think of myself as an anxious person. I'm not an excessive worrier. I'm not shy. I can get up in front of a crowd or talk down the barrel of a TV camera without breaking a sweat. Someone like me couldn't possibly have anxiety.

The birth of my first daughter, Esther, four years ago, was followed by a series of challenging events. I went back to work soon after she was born, to a stressful and public role as a Member of Parliament. Determined to breastfeed, I was pumping around the clock, expressing between caucus meetings and select committee hearings, feeling as though I was being torn in two every time I left her. She was not a good sleeper and I was chronically sleep-deprived. Meanwhile my partner, Dave, who had taken time off work to be her primary caregiver, developed chronic pain and was unable to continue looking after her full-time. I took on the bulk of the domestic work. Things started to feel very hard. It became clear that I couldn't continue as an MP, so after battling it out for six months I stepped down. The pressure eased a little, but the damage was done. I had severe postnatal anxiety.

My anxiety does not look like worrying. It looks like indecision, paralysis, agitation and, if poorly managed, rage and self-harm. But it is still anxiety. I've spent much of the last four years coming to understand this. It's a strange thing, having to revise your ideas about yourself. For me, it has meant learning, over and over, that I have a new set of limitations. I am an accomplished, high-achieving person. I used to pack a lot into a day. I had an accurate sense of what I was capable of, and I could almost always say yes to a request or an opportunity. Now, every decision weighs heavily on me. Can I write this essay? Can I manage this social engagement? Can I prepare this meal?

When Esther was a toddler there were things I desperately wished I could do with her, but which fear and indecision kept me from. I had visions of her playing happily in the sand at Petone Beach, dipping her toes in, exploring her local environment. Instead I trudged up and down the path parallel to the beach with her asleep in the buggy, watching families with picnic blankets, packets of fish and chips, beers, kites and swimsuits, apparently carefree. Dave was at home in pain, with no desire to go anywhere near the beach. If I wanted it to happen, it was my job. But every time I thought about it, I became overwhelmed with all the risks I'd have to manage and the gear I'd need to take with me. I told myself we'd go another day.

These days it's easier to get to the beach, but simple things still elude me, like enjoying downtime when I get it. It feels like time passes differently for me than for other people. Hours seem to slip through my fingers as I fret, paralysed with indecision about where to start on the long list of things I could or should be doing. The world jangles. There's a cacophony of sound. I am compelled to turn off household noise—TV, extractor fan, music. I walk into a cluttered and messy room (which is often all the rooms of my house) and feel overwhelmed. But the indecision about what to do first stops me from restoring order, so I can't reclaim the space, either. I delay, and put on a podcast, or perhaps run a bath. I could justify these things as acts of self-care, intentional relaxation, but I can't stop thinking about the mess I should be cleaning or the words I should be writing. What should be restorative simply eats up my time—and then here everyone comes, back already.

My anxiety makes it difficult for me to spend time alone with my daughter. I love her, and when I'm not with her I miss her. Yet faced with a few hours of unstructured time together, I panic. She has an unquenchable thirst for my attention, which makes simple household tasks like cooking feel near impossible. She'll make so many demands of me. She'll mess up the house. She'll yell at me from another room. Or she'll insist on helping and break something or hurt herself. Often, she is defiant and challenging. Thinking ahead, I'll plan an activity that will get us out of the house together, like a trip to a playground or the library, but sometimes she just really needs to be at home. In these agitated times, I rely on the stupefying distraction of screen time to get us through until Dave arrives home. Then I feel guilty about that.

In recent months I've thought a lot about whether to medicate for my anxiety. Several friends have described to me the feeling of going on anti-anxiety or antidepressant medications for the first time: the quieting of the cacophony of sound in their heads, the end of intrusive or unhelpful thoughts, the wonder—is this how everyone else feels all the time? I want that feeling.

Yet I haven't discussed medication with any health professionals. Whenever I get close, I am stopped by the same thought: this shouldn't be so hard. My conviction that the answer lies not in mitigating individual circumstances, but in changing the societal conditions that create them, stops me from accessing the help I probably need. There's a circularity and futility in this, I know.

I lay my experience of becoming a mother alongside my grandmother's. So much has changed for women in 60 years. Law changes emphasising civil rights, pay equity and financial and legal independence. Social changes like the widespread availability of contraception, the creation of childcare options and the expectation that women will work after marriage. Second-wave feminism, debunking the myths of gender essentialism. Increasing proportions of women in leadership roles across society (though by no means enough). Paid parental leave, and the understanding that this can be shared by both parents. Much better knowledge of mental illness and how to treat it.

But the similarities between my experience and Lucy's are undeniable, connecting us across the years. The sudden shock of motherhood. Loss of professional identity. Caring for an unwell partner. Feeling like you are doing it all on your own. Despite all that has changed for women in the intervening years, these remain common experiences.

The woman in the archival film clip, stuck at home with her baby, longing for the company of men and women, thought work might be the answer. Now it is easier for mothers to re-enter the workforce, but we are still suffering. The incidence of perinatal anxiety and depression in New Zealand is currently estimated at around 25 percent.

I think many of the changes that have empowered women to seek experiences and careers beyond the domestic sphere have perpetuated the myth that we can do so with ease, *at the same time* as parenting, running a household and upholding care responsibilities. Rather than addressing the gender role assumptions and valuing and sharing this workload, we have simply added to the expectations placed on our grandmothers. Most mothers I know feel compelled, whether by financial necessity or societal expectation, to fulfil the roles of both the domestic and the working woman. Many struggle with anxiety, guilt, depression, exhaustion. Many medicate. All wish it were easier.

A few weeks after completing the first draft of this essay, I gave birth to my second daughter, Ngaire. The birth was fast, crazy and exhilarating, and I found myself on a high for months afterwards. My anxiety receded. Unwelcome thoughts quietened, and I viewed the chaos of family life with a mixture of humour and resignation. My parenting decisions were not governed by fear, but by a strong conviction that all would be well. I found the feeling I'd been craving, the sense of calm and normalcy.

As the months have passed and the relentlessness of life with a baby and a preschooler has set in, some anxiety has returned. My new limitations are still there; I know this is likely something I'll have to actively manage for the rest of my life. But I've thought a lot about what my second postnatal experience means for this essay, in which I've wondered about not just what might help to ease individual circumstances, but also what might help to reduce the overall incidence of maternal anxiety and distress. It feels significant to me that this time I felt no expectation or pressure to return to work. I had high quality early childhood education for my older daughter, meals delivered by kind family members and friends for weeks after the birth, and access to a psychologist.

Paid parental leave. Subsidised early childhood education. Community support and connection. Access to mental health services. Some of these things I received by right, or by the generosity of others. Some of them I paid for. Some are near impossible for most women to access without financial support or long, long waiting lists. All were essential.

Lucy died eight years ago, aged 92. She had a long and fulfilling life, but I was sad that she didn't get to see me enter Parliament nor meet her great-granddaughters, one of whom carries her name. When she was alive she would tell me the same stories a lot: stories about her working life, the tennis parties, the dances and the scary times resuscitating my grandfather. Not so much about her experiences parenting small children. I wasn't yet a parent myself, so I never thought to ask her why she didn't really talk about that part of her life. Now I wish I could. What was it really like to be Mrs Housewife in the suburbs in the 1950s? How did she get through the hard days? What would she have changed?

The Curse Machine

Kate Kennedy

The day I secretly conducted a sacred burial service for my elderly relatives' African mask was the day I knew that anxiety—panic, terror, call it what you will—had destroyed me. I thought it was cursed; I thought *I* was cursed. There I was, up in the bush on my knees in the dirt, spraying aromatherapy oils around the place and chanting God knows what over what was most likely a benign gift-shop souvenir. I was 25 years old, and my head—along with my world—had exploded.

Though it took years for my anxiety and panic to escalate to the point where I thought a souvenir was out to get me, the signs had been there for a while. I can recall a handful of incidents from childhood where I flipped out beyond a normal spectrum of fear.

The first panic attack I remember was the day I got my foot stuck in a raft made out of a wooden pallet. My jammed foot dangled in the water while my brother on the bank shouted, 'The eels'll get ya!' I screamed at levels unheard of in our sleepy street. As a child and young teenager I had no name for the overpowering emotion that would flood my brain, my body, all my circuitry and wiring. But anxiety, fear and panic were an ambush on constant standby.

If I were a young person today I would probably be observed, assessed, counselled, medicated and generally bubble-wrapped (assuming our creaking mental health services could find the space). But in the 1970s and early 1980s, the gold-standard strategies for dealing with anxious children were something like: shut them alone in detention rooms, humiliate them, send them to boarding school, ground them, blame them for not pulling themselves together, shout at them a lot. It's unfathomable how far we've come. A Google search for 'students and anxiety' today gets 228 million results; as a high-school student growing up anxious in 1981, I never even saw a book about it.

So I found my own treatments. I started off smoking cigarettes which I stole from my dad, but it wasn't long before I discovered the highs and lows of binge-drinking and smoking pot. Older students were always willing to supply the alcohol, and cannabis was prevalent in my town, too. We scored it at parties, and kids stole it from their parents. It wasn't hard to find. When I was getting drunk or high—or both—I had a good time. Think parties, adventures, reckless thrills; getting wasted was relaxing and distracting. Emotionally, there was definitely a powerful 'pull factor' of escapism. Being straight and stuck in my own head? Not so much. My parents' marriage was breaking apart, I was constantly in trouble for being a bored, misbehaving kid in the classroom, I was trying to keep secret the fact that I might be a lesbian, and there was an undercurrent of darkness in my life that I was not yet consciously aware of—that I had been sexually abused as a child. These circumstances were pushing and pulling my mind and my behaviour in every direction. In hindsight, it is no surprise that I was struggling to cope and self-medicating at every available opportunity.

University was a tough change of gear, and the stress of academic study was compounded by my unacknowledged, untreated, seismic capacity for anxiety. I was an applied student during my first two years. I didn't smoke much weed over this time, mainly just at student parties, so I felt every little bit of that stress. By now it was the mid 1980s. Still there was no awareness of mental health, no public campaign and no sympathy from those in positions of power. I remember going to see one of my lecturers to ask for an extension on an assignment. I was in tears, stressed to the max. In between sobs, I pleaded for an extension. She stared me down. I don't remember her words, exactly, but the message was clear: toughen up and get on with it or you will never make it here. I thought I would snap.

Once again I found a way to escape the pressure when I made my way back to cannabis in the late 1980s. I'd found a new tribe, and with them I rediscovered the calming social effects of marijuana. We were totally ignorant of the effects of regular cannabis use on people with mental health issues and relied exclusively on information transmitted either from our friends ('pot is great') or from parents ('pot paves the road to hell'). There was no middle ground. But when it comes to cannabis, what can be a good time or a good medicine for one person can create a ticking time bomb in another. While I was hanging out with my friends, smoking dope, listening to Bob Marley and Pink Floyd on rotate, chilling out and reducing my stress, somewhere deep inside my brain a kind of chemistry was starting to react. I was blissfully unaware, and continued to smoke. It worked for me—until it didn't.

The results were catastrophic: at age 24, a severe episode of psychosis (where those African masks would not shut up) which took several psychiatric hospital admissions and years of psychiatric medication to place in remission; surfaced memories of childhood sexual abuse, the genesis of a lifetime of PTSD. At 26, after more ill-advised drug use, including a brain-busting foray into magic mushrooms, the explosion of my anxiety into a clinically identifiable panic disorder that almost destroyed my life.

A sane person would have stopped using there, but sanity had well and truly left the building. Somewhere along this ruinous path, I had become addicted to cannabis. I couldn't cope with the day unless my mind was numb; I was convinced that the power of what lay on the other side of that fog would put me in my grave.

I had no awareness of this descent into addiction. If you'd tried to tell me, I would say mind your own business, and not that politely. But what everyone could see was that my attempts at coping were turning me into a paranoid shadow. I'd become so reliant that I believed that cannabis was keeping me alive. I'd dropped out of life, existing on a benefit, and my stints between hospital admissions were characterised by returning time and again to the people who could give me drugs. I smoked cannabis with them, and then more frequently on my own. I resented having to spend time with friends or family who didn't smoke weed, as it got in the way of my using. I was terrified of getting busted for possession. I crept in and out of dealers' houses, certain I was being watched, and combined with my PTSD I was jumping at every shadow. I thought cars were following me, I believed that the community psych team was tracking me, and that the police were bugging my phone. I felt driven, obsessed and possessed.

Those of us who smoked a lot didn't see ourselves as addicts. We saw ourselves as somehow superior, and looked down from our holy pinnacles at the madness of the world and the tedium of people who didn't smoke. In reality, our collective mental health was in shreds.

To be honest, I never really grasped the whole anxiety–cannabis–addiction matrix until I was admitted to a psychiatric hospital, one of so many invisible young people who have disappeared into that particular Bermuda Triangle. Paradoxically, the admission came about because I'd tried to stop smoking weed after my first psychotic meltdown and flashbacks. Once I had nothing to manage and mask my depression and anxiety, the totality of my inner terror came crashing through those walls which I had unconsciously constructed and then hastily torn down. I couldn't sleep. I jumped at shadows. I heard voices telling me evil, Satanic things. I thought—no, I knew—I was possessed, and I started to lose my grip on reality. If I'd been told then that I had an anxiety disorder, I would have scoffed at the pettiness of the word. Anxiety? But I was living in total fear and dread 24/7, and my biggest source of terror was that I would wake tomorrow and it would all be the same. For a terrible time in my life, it was.

Now the early 90s, still there was little official recognition of the link between cannabis use and diminished mental wellbeing. Of course, the doctors in the psychiatric hospital were aware of the link because so many of their patients smoked a lot of cannabis. Today those patients would be considered addicts, particularly those referred to as the 'revolving door' clientele. But it wasn't until 2013 that the conditions of cannabis-induced anxiety disorder and cannabis-induced insomnia were officially recognised in the profession's 'bible', the *Diagnostic and Statistical Manual of Mental Disorders*. At the time I was in hospital, doctors didn't have a lot of tools to work with, mainly just a limited and outdated pharmaceutical arsenal with roughly the equivalent medical clout of being drowned in a bucket of mud. This meant that, eventually, if I was to find my way out of this maze of admissions, relapses and readmissions, I was going to have to find some other way of dealing with this inexplicable barrage of emotions which were literally driving me crazy.

Thank god I eventually found recovery. I'd ventured into the rooms of Narcotics Anonymous (NA) a few times in the course of my addiction madness, on the suggestion of wiser friends and health professionals, but I'd never managed to stay long. I just couldn't stay clean—I had been unable to accept that I couldn't use drugs or alcohol again. Because how on earth would I survive my anxiety, my intense fear and pain, without the numbness? I'd even tried rehab, but my frail, PTSD-riddled mind could not cope with sharing rooms with strangers, and after a short time I had bolted. But at age 33 I showed up at an NA meeting an exhausted, tear-stained, shaking mess. I had simply nowhere else left to go, and at least I had witnessed the presence of hope in those rooms before, and a possibility of a sense of future unlike what I had seen in the hospital and other mental health services, where many of the same people went around and around in the maze until they took their own lives. I knew I had to get through this. So I went to NA ostensibly to deal with my cannabis addiction, for which by now there was incontrovertible evidence, a crisis even I could not ignore, that I was living a half-life as a numbed-out trainwreck.

NA meetings are similar to how you see them on TV: a group of people sit in a room taking turns to share their experiences of what happened to them and how they were able to change. But what TV fails to capture is the feeling in the room, the wairua or spirit of those powerful stories, connections and transformations. Through that wairua, I was able to find not only recovery from drugs, but a glimpse of freedom from my barely suppressed inner turmoil. I came to see that I could be free from the fear and anxiety that had driven my reactions, poor decisions and patterns of behaviour from a very young age. Other people, just like me, had found peace.

But first, I had to admit that I was beaten. Like, really admit it. I had to accept that everything I had tried prior to this moment had failed to equip me with the resilience and resources to handle my life circumstances and the way those made me feel. I had to accept that using drugs was never going to be an adequate solution, that they would never make me better. I had to close the door completely on my drug and alcohol use all the way this time, not leaving ajar that little crack of reservation, as I had done on my previous attempts. I had to be willing to change.

I'd never previously succeeded at staying clean, but this time was different. On some visceral level I understood that I had to face some facts. Being stoned was no longer containing my anxiety; it was fuelling it. Instead of becoming calm, lately when I smoked I felt paranoid and stressed. I would get headaches or feel the walls were closing in. And yet when I would stop or ease up on my intake, I would feel cranky, restless and unhappy. I couldn't live with my remedy and I couldn't live without it. I was ready to accept step one of the NA programme: I was powerless over my addiction (and my mental state) and my life had become unmanageable. Unexpectedly, I immediately felt an incredible sense of peace and relief, and so I stayed. Peace and relief had been all I'd ever wanted, I just hadn't know it till then.

The 12 steps of the Anonymous programmes (Alcoholics Anonymous, Narcotics Anonymous and the myriad of other addiction programmes that have sprung up under that banner) contain the most remarkable and practical means to achieve healing and inner peace that I have encountered—and believe me, I've tried a few things. Through studying the 12 steps and participating in NA and other 12-step fellowship meetings, I've experienced vital and transformative realisations about who I am as a person, how I work, and how I came to be a prisoner to emotional and psychological trauma. Most importantly, the fearless self-examination encouraged by these programmes has enabled me to make better choices for my future than the ones I can now see I made in the past.

One of the first things I learned was to put myself in context, because while I couldn't say how I ended up in this dark place, I blamed myself. I learned how addiction is a survival mechanism, unconsciously chosen though a dysfunctional method of dealing with pain. I can honour that addiction got me through—drugs worked, to a point, but to a point where I could no longer ignore my pain. It was either move forward or jump off.

I knew I needed to change, and this seemed a scarier proposition than it actually turned out to be. In itself, this illustrated anxiety to me: I was looking at life through a lens of fear, an emotion I was applying to every situation. I learned how to change that perception. I can choose to apply another lens through which to view the ever-changing circumstances that life presents me with. I can free myself from fear. Becoming conscious of my 'fear lens' was probably the most liberating realisation I had in my recovery.

The second most liberating realisation, and this one came later, was how hard I was on myself. I had this tape playing in my head that I had no conscious awareness of. It contained a voice that criticised me constantly and mercilessly, telling me I wasn't good enough, that I was a failure who didn't deserve happiness or peace. The discovery of the tape and the 'fear lens' explained the basis of much of my dysfunctional thinking and behaviour. No wonder I was anxious!

I had unmasked these malevolent malfunctions for the total frauds that they really were. Knowledge gave me the power to decide to do things differently, to start speaking to myself with kindness and care, to try to look at day-to-day events as opportunities for growth and change, and maybe even through which to find happiness. I had to deprogramme my fear response and replace it with a baby-steps version of faith. When I catch myself thinking 'What if I've left the oven on and the house burns down?'(even though I checked it three times before I went out), I override it with a different message, like 'Everything is okay.' When I find myself getting anxious over what is happening in somebody else's life, I practise 'detaching with love' from that person. When I'm freaking out at three in the morning, thinking 'What if I have cancer?' I replace that thought with 'What if I don't?'.

I'm not saying I'm fully at peace with my anxiety yet, but I look back to where I came from and think, 'If I can get well, anybody can.' For me, the whole way that I viewed life and the perception I had of myself needed a serious overhaul. But the outcome—the experience of faith, trust, serenity and the acceptance of happiness—has brought about a simple life more fulfilling than anything I could have imagined.

I've been clean and sober for over 17 years now, and I am grateful for every single day of triumph over self-destruction that I have found through the 12 steps. The tyranny of fear that consumed me seems like a surreal, long-ago nightmare, leaving a healed-over scar that reminds me daily how great it is to be free. I couldn't do it alone, though. To recover myself, I had to find other people who knew how to get there. And I recommend that you do, too.

Worry People

Madeline Reid

It has been a long time since I've been to see a therapist and, now, I am going to see a woman called Vivienne. Before we meet I picture her in purple dungarees, with straw-coloured hair and two children in the back of a Subaru. I picture her in a Grey Lynn villa, cultivating her own garden and living life slowly. Vivienne costs just 30 dollars a month and, in the daily grind of panic and my 60-hour work weeks, I tell myself once a month is enough. For a first-year teacher, it's an achievable amount of time in an endlessly busy life.

The first time I knock on her door under its wreath of bougainvillea, catching a whiff of incense, I have this underwater feeling of dread. I've forgotten how to cherry-pick the parts of my illness, the best parts that can be spoken about to a counsellor, neat and ready for consumption. I think about how to phrase things delicately. You see, I can tell someone about the meltdowns—that's easy. I can tell you how on the same day I was accepted into my Master's degree I was assessed by an emergency mental health team at Cornwall House. I can tell you that if you take enough antipsychotics, they will grind your muscles into parcels of sand, or that I did my best work at Pak'nSave while on Valium, and spent my 21st birthday with my family of sentries, nursing me in bed. But I can't tell people about the voices I hear, and disclose what it is they demand.

Vivienne offers me tea, but my neck is too stiff to drink it without shaking. She asks me how a functional voice-hearer with chronic anxiety has managed to get through teachers' training.

'I push myself too hard all the time,' I say. 'I can't tell if that's just how my life is now, or if I'm supposed to be giving myself a rest, or something.'

My stockings are unkempt and laddered. I haven't washed my hair in a week, and I let this feeling follow me—casting my eyes down—burning and ashamed.

'There's something political in that,' she says. 'In the tenor of your voice. A sort of defiance, as it were.'

'I don't think I'm political,' I say. 'I don't sit on the motorway with signs. I don't really protest.'

'This is a different kind of protest,' she says, and I stop asking questions, because I don't know what she means by that.

She taps her nails on the edge of her laptop. 'So you've identified that you would like to learn how to accept uncertainty, and embrace the uncertainty of the future. But what does this look like for you? What do you envisage happening?'

I think that the past looks too heavy to mention. It reminds me of squeezing my toes under seats in lecture theatres, straining my shoulder and locking my jaw and twitching whenever a tutor asked me a question. It reminds me of a physical, sweaty ungodliness and fretting in coffee queues, of running out of a public restaurant crying and throwing up between my legs. Cowering under the piano during a music lesson, with all of the other students writing away and feeling normal things like wishing they were somewhere else. My heart was beating so fast I went to the GP the next day to get my thyroid checked. The past is calling out for my mother in tears and accidentally screaming, Take me to hospital, I'm dying, I'm dying, then she's pinning me down in her room. That's the thing with my anxiety: whenever it returns, it's always something different—with variation and substance, daring and style. It keeps me on my toes.

But anxiety has also taught me things, like about the nature of fear. It has left me unable to shower, get out of bed or respond to a question in under a minute. It has kept me away from school and university, locked in a room with water-marked magazines and oppressive air conditioning and a psychiatrist who's practised in knowing a safe distance, who knows the right moment to let a smile break across her face.

I remember every doctor I have ever seen and the manner in which they have spoken to me. How they used to beam at my parents and pat my shoulder and say, You, Madeline Reid, *you* are going to be a success story one day. The way they said it made me think there must not be many success stories out there, for them to go on and on like this. Perhaps I would be one for the collection. Even now, if I bring up the past and its trauma, my mother will say to me, But you are a success story, Madeline. There's not many like you out there!

The youth mental-health system doesn't exactly set you up for success. After a few years of trying different methods and medications, I began to make little self-addressed envelopes. Some had chocolate in them and others had little messages that read: I am enough, I do enough, I'm good enough. I'd hide them around the house to find by accident. More recently, my mother painted a homemade die so that I could throw it whenever I was frightened and it would tell me what to do. One side read: take a bath. Another: make a cup of tea. Another: read your book. But it couldn't stop the unpredictable panic episodes, running down Kohimarama Road screaming because I thought a stranger was going to hurt me. Nor could it stop me from quitting on anyone who ever invited me out because I assumed they wouldn't like me. I've learnt that antipsychotics don't rewrite my thought patterns, and cognitive behavioural therapy can't transform my learned behaviours. There's just time and light, and the unfortunate things that happen in between. And for many years, too many things were happening in between.

In the staffroom where I teach, the principal often starts morning briefings with discussions on student anxiety. They aren't coping with the demands of the world—social media, lack of financial security, rises in unemployment, and the fallacy of perfection. I have been drilled to follow correct procedure when a student has a panic attack, and I have to bite my tongue to stop myself from saying, 'Oh yes—just last week I nearly went to hospital with one of those!' or 'I know how it is. I've been in and out of the system for eight years.' I have to stop myself from feeling sick or from dwelling on the question at the bottom of my employment contract: *Do you live with any physical/mental health condition that might impact your ability to do this job safely?*

There is an acknowledged stigma against having any sort of mental illness. This stigma tells me that, because I have anxiety, I can't cope with it. And yet, the defiant act of coping can break the foundations of that stigma. I have not disclosed to my colleagues that I suffer from a variety-basket of conditions, and I feel that if I did, they would either fire me or exercise a sudden disbelief. When I've told people in the past, they've often become unsure of me—because I don't behave in the expected manner of someone anxious and out of touch with reality, and it makes them wary. Some wear their honesty like a medal and voice their reactions tactlessly, referring to me as insane, batshit and unstable. One even said of me, 'She is a dark person, who has attracted dark things to her.' What is it about mental illness that makes people think it's a choice? If people could pick their failures in romance, success and health, there would be fewer repeat prescriptions for sale. Chemists everywhere would give up their jobs, psychiatrists would return to university.

There is still a tension between feeling as though I'm a productive person, capable of handling a busy teaching job, and then feeling as though I won't make registration after two years, because you're only allowed so many sick days. All of it comes down to this barrier. I learned about this word—barrier—at university during a lecture on adolescent mental health. The lecturer talked about depression, anxiety, bipolar disorder and nothing else. It's easy to contribute to the erasure of psychosis from mental-health discussions—it happens often, as more palatable conditions take the stage. But I stared at the projector and felt this quote resonate with me: 'Disability is a process which happens when one group of people create barriers by designing a world only for their way of living.'

'Barriers' continued to follow me around. During my first high-school placement I met with a lecturer who had come to observe my lesson. We were sitting in a drab fish-bowl of a conference room when she shut the 60-page handbook and turned to me. 'Do you have a disability?' she asked.

I answered with the same uneasiness I used to feel when I had just come out as gay, and my peers would ask me which female celebrities I found attractive. 'Yes,' I said carefully. 'I do. Sort of. But it's not the kind that will get in the way of my teaching.'

'Two sick days,' she frowned, scanning my teaching log. 'What happened there?'

I told her it was because of migraines.

'Well, you'll have to be careful,' she said. 'If you miss more than five days on your practicum, you'll have to repeat it.'

I tell Vivienne that I've dealt with chronic illness like I've dealt with every other difficult thing in my life—in daily ministrations, where the smaller things are part of a bigger thing, where nothing is the biggest, best or worst. There is never a perfect month, I tell her. *Vivienne, darling, there is never a calm week.* Each year is riddled with hindrances which I speak to very few people about. Pulling over on a dual carriageway and nesting my head in my hands. Dropping a tube of toothpaste and flinching at an unexpected voice in my head saying, 'Pick that up.' Trying to eat at a potluck without hyperventilating.

Hiding far away from the others, with their jokes and their drinks and each other, losing it at the sheer breadth of noise in my head. In each of these instances I feel the distance between me and everything else, and it is the kind which cannot be breached.

'We keep coming back to this thing,' Vivienne says, 'this distance. You feel it between yourself and others. Between reality and panic, and a loss of personal control.'

'Yes,' I say.

It's true, I'm afraid of losing control. The feeling of losing control is the first symptom of a panic attack, and the thing that lingers with you many years after you've had a psychotic episode. It doesn't come in the form of worried afterthoughts; it's a long, stewing permeation. For those of us who lose control over our thoughts, emotions and perceptions, there is something uniquely liberating about recognising this lack of control and acknowledging the space between stability and instability. It's almost restorative, because we begin to recognise the privilege of every moment in which we do have control, and we begin to harness these.

I cannot sleep. My mother has put these South American dolls she calls 'worry people' under my pillow, but still I cannot sleep. I arrive at school at quarter to seven and traipse down the spine of the courtyard into the cramped halls of S-Block. H-Block is where we normally teach English, but the roof had been leaking and then caved in, and the principal is in a war with the ministry about it. The lights are always off or flickering. I'm the first to turn them on. Dry ice and smoke plumes out from the resource room, where stacks of paper and old textbooks line the benches. My heart is already thumping too fast because I've had too much coffee, to try and boost my alertness for the day ahead. Recently one of my students turned on the gas taps in class and, since then, whenever I feel the one o'clock drowsiness descending, I start to panic that if I close my eyes I won't wake up again. In the hallway, the usual earlybirds smile and nod. I have noticed that the closer we get to holidays, the harder those smiles get. Even the most veteran teachers feel they must hide their stress or fear they might be seen as weak for getting the butterflies before a tough class—Year 10s on a Friday afternoon, or in the library, or anywhere.

At times, when I've dissociated and muddled up some of my favourite students' names or incorrectly taught a metaphor, I've felt about to faint. I've looked down at my hands and felt cut off from my body.

Then there are the moments of catharsis. Recently, I've begun investing $80 a term on an hour-long massage. I come out with the cold rush of relief one feels after finishing an exam, the same spring in my step that I see in my students as they race down the halls for the holiday break. I find catharsis, the release of fear and inadequacy and how others might view me, in the small acts of these students: the boy who refused to sit quietly but will now write in silence in my classes; the students who smile and wave, who bring me words and lollies and worries, and I begin to feel a strange sense of pride swelling my chest.

Now, in my eighth year of chronic illness, I am pacing ahead in strides. They are not always even, but at least they're moving in the right direction. When I was younger and stumbling, I used to think I had too many tough experiences for my age and not enough life to catch up to them. But lately I have been feeling like life is catching up, and I would like it, in whatever bright and profound and disastrous way it will, to continue. Whether it's through scheduled visits to a counsellor or in psychiatric medicine or the use of narrative therapy, I would like it to continue.

I don't believe in revelations, recovery or answers. There's no lightbulb that smashes into tiny halogen pieces. Only in books do people have the time to pause and think of original ways to react to something. In life, and with any kind of mental illness or anxiousness, you're not allowed to sit and wallow in it like in an armchair on a long afternoon, and wait for it to pass while the whole world sinks around you. Some things can't be processed; some things can't be hidden, like the marks my damp palms leave on a student's desk. I am supposed to be the mother hen and the figure of authority, a form of protection, even, and a form of guidance. But I am still trying to protect myself. This is the first time I acknowledge this fact, at the end of an hour-long session on a work night.

Vivienne tells me that our time is up and asks me to fill out an evaluation form. It is my second meeting with her and the company are already getting me to assess her performance.

'A functional voice-hearer,' she says, as she holds the door ajar. The scent of autumn and the misty garden coasts through. The Auckland sky is washed pink and grey, and the rain has begun to fall.

'You have given yourself this term, haven't you Madeline? You have gifted it,' she continues, pushing the hinges out of their sockets, ever further. 'You have gifted it to yourself.'

Scared to Death

Kerry Sunderland

The summit of Whitehorn Pass is a permanent ice field. I am watching some sort of weird headless stick-insect crunch its way across the glacier. It is my husband, David, wearing crampons. All I can see are two thin pale legs below the old-school green and purple canvas backpack he has retrieved from our attic. He normally takes his modern, lightweight pack, but it wouldn't fit all the food he needed to carry on this six-day tramp across three mountain passes in the Southern Alps.

Then, as swiftly as a thin envelope slips into the top of a postbox, I watch him disappear. The ice has gobbled him up. There are two very tall members of his tramping party—Sylvan, dressed in a bright red cowboy hat and silky blue boxer-shorts emblazoned with the New Zealand flag, and Dwarf, who describes himself as 'a skinny guy on stilts'. They lie on their stomachs and reach over the infinity edge of the concave waterfall, but cannot reach him.

I exhale deeply. I am not there. I did not see my husband eaten by ice. I am in bed, and I have merely imagined it.

It's late summer and a few days ago I left David and five of our friends on the western side of Klondyke Corner to start the tramp. Now I am home again and, just before bed, I read that when the sun is shining after heavy rain, steep crevasses can develop on Whitehorn Pass. I've checked the rainfall and 247 millimetres has fallen in the area over the past seven days.

Somehow, I know that the crevasses are almost impossible to see until you're on top of them.

I exhale deeply. I am guessing it's about three o'clock in the morning and I've been awake for what feels like hours.

I'm trying to fill my mind with rational arguments, to stop the scene replaying in my mind. But all I can feel is fear, as amorphous and infinite as this dark moonless night. I realise I am holding my breath. I exhale deeply. I exhale deeply again. And again.

Eventually, I can feel the steady rhythm has returned. Not long after, I slip into a deep slumber until our rooster, Mr Gilderoy, greets the first light.

A few hours later, I wake and find myself weighed down with an anxiety hangover. Since my visits from anxiety are typically nocturnal, I know these type of hangovers well—the deep exhaustion mixed with embarrassment and, if I'm lucky, the essence of relief. Somehow, between those long hours awake with worry and the alarm going off, I must have fallen asleep.

When I tell my friends I'm feeling anxious because my husband has set off on a difficult tramp only a few days after ex-Cyclone Fehi hit the West Coast, they reassure me it's not unreasonable. When I tell them I'm feeling anxious when David's gone hunting, they also reassure me. They don't say, 'You've got nothing to worry about'; they tell me it's a reasonable fear. But whether or not the fear of *what might happen* is reasonable or unreasonable matters little to me. The physical effects are the same, even when the circumstances might be unreasonable. I can still feel my heartbeat vibrate through me. I can hear nothing other than my churchbell-volume pulse. I feel like I'm drowning in a sea of oxygen. Someone is winding up a winch to extract the muscles in my legs out of an imaginary hole in my lower abdomen.

Occasional bouts of anxiety are normal. Technically, they become an anxiety disorder when they do not go away. In my experience, anxiety feeds on anxiety. Without any effort on my part, it can soon become a bloated creature, a bit like a goldfish with dropsy that's been turfed into the toilet but won't flush away and is left bobbing amongst the detritus, its wee mouth appearing to gasp for breath. One of the main symptoms of anxiety, insomnia, also means it's really easy to get stuck in the toilet bowl. All of a sudden, I am consumed by anxious thoughts about simple everyday happenings. For me, already having lost one mate in this lifetime, the anxiety can often be fixated. I feel anxious when David's driving home from work after a long day. I feel anxious when he's clearing the gutters. I feel anxious when he uses insect spray. I don't verbalise this anxiety because I know how silly it is. I don't want to wrap my husband in energetic cotton wool, so I subconsciously gravitate towards opportunities to be distracted and disconnected. The upshot of this is that I can't sleep, find it difficult to get out of bed in the morning, convince myself that I am too busy to exercise, too busy to make myself a decent meal—and too wound up even to phone a friend. You can't cheat on anxiety; emotions are stored in the body before they become conscious thoughts. This loop continues indefinitely, until I attempt to control my thoughts—to stop *worrying about the future*—by focussing my awareness on the simplest of things: am I holding my breath?

Researchers have found genetic and environmental risk factors for anxiety disorder. I can tick many of these boxes. I am female, I have been widowed, I was exposed to stressful events in my childhood and, just last year, was locked in a house against my will. There is a history of mental illness in my family. I haven't had my saliva tested, but there's a good chance I have elevated cortisol levels in the afternoons. Most people experience a mid-afternoon crash when their cortisol, the primary stress-response hormone, drops, but those with anxiety often don't. Excess cortisol in the afternoons causes a hair-trigger response to stress, and sleep problems. Knowing this has made me vigilant when it comes to ensuring I take a break for a half-hour walk along the beach or in the forest at the end of every work day.

Joe Dispenza, a writer and researcher who has focussed on the intersection between neuroscience, epigenetics and quantum physics, notes that a series of highly charged, emotionally stressful events within a short time frame have the potential to switch on the body's stress response. When the stress response can't be turned off, one effectively lives in survival mode, an energetic 'state of emergency'.

> Here is where things can go from bad to worse. In preparation for the next perceived threat, a person will think about some future worst-case scenario—based on a specific past memory—and will emotionally embrace it with such focus and concentration, that their body begins to believe that it is living in that future reality in the present moment. Why? Because the body is the unconscious mind. It does not know the difference between an actual experience in life that creates an emotion or when an emotion is created by thought alone. As a result, the body can get knocked out of homeostasis just by thinking.[1]

When I was child, I suffered panic attacks but didn't know what they were. They were characterised by shortness of breath and the feeling of being trapped in a loop of emotions and fearful thoughts.

When I look back, I can pretty much pinpoint the arrival of anxiety in my life. It hitched a ride with its co-conspirator, the fear of death. My father was obsessed with aviation and flew gliders competitively, so much of my childhood was spent on dusty Australian gliding fields, developing a subterranean fear that he would vanish from the sky. Most weekends, my parents made the four-hour return roadtrip from the southeastern suburbs of Melbourne to the local gliding field in Bacchus Marsh, where I was part of a large tribe of gliding kids who looked after themselves all day and sometimes well into the

---

1 Joe Dispenza, 'The Anatomy of Anxiety', *Dr Joe Dispenza's Blog*, n.d. drjoedispenza.com/blog/health/the-anatomy-of-anxiety/

evening. I coped with any sense of abandonment by reading, almost pathologically, seeking out surrogate families wherever I could, and disappearing inside my imagination, but even that didn't assuage the fear. It wasn't entirely unreasonable, since in the small Australian gliding community in the 1970s, there seemed to me to be a disproportionately high number of fatal gliding accidents. The first I remember was Lois Piggott, who had befriended me at a gliding camp in Benalla. I would climb up on to an enormous wooden stool in Lois's kitchen and chat to her while I ate biscuits. She was warm and friendly and I loved spending time with her. One day her glider literally fell out of the sky over Bacchus Marsh. Her death is the first I really felt, somewhere deep in my body.

It was ironic that my anxiety about the death of loved ones manifested in breathing difficulties. From an early age, I struggled with breathing. I could never complete the long-distance run at school without hyperventilating. I had trouble sleeping in unfamiliar surroundings, and would lie awake gasping for air. Soon I started to develop patterns or habits in a bid to create, as Karl Ove Knausgård writes, a 'framework or scaffolding around the unpredictable'.[2] These routines and rituals included obsessive hand-washing and a tendency to be risk-averse by proxy, while wildly disregarding my own wellbeing and safety.

The breathing problems that plagued me throughout my childhood were finally diagnosed as asthma when I was in my final year of secondary school. In my mid 20s, I was twice hospitalised as a result of severe asthma attacks. If you can't breathe properly, it's really easy to be anxious.

In my early 30s, I met my first husband, Steve, a traditional Chinese medicine practitioner and *taiji* (tai chi) teacher. He first taught me how to breathe using the ancient Chinese practice of *qi gong*. For thousands of years, the Chinese have studied how

---

[2] *Winter: Seasons Quartet 2* (Random House, 2017), 'Fireworks', Kindle.

energy flows through the human body, along a transportation system of 'meridians' (channels) that often run in parallel with the cardiovascular system. They call this energy *qi* (pronounced 'chee'); sometimes it's defined as air or breath, but really it means 'life force' or 'vital essence'—so *qi gong* roughly translates as 'internal energy work'. Practising *qi gong* ensures energy doesn't get blocked in the transportation network. Steve also started treating me with Chinese herbs, acupuncture and moxibustion. Basically, Chinese medicine sees asthma as a three-part condition involving bronchial constriction, inflammation and plugs of mucous, all of which needed to be treated in different ways. In Chinese terms, the bronchial constriction is related to 'liver chi stagnation' and is treated with acupuncture. Chinese herbs can treat the inflammation and tonify the spleen, which can resolve the damp and phlegm for the mucous condition. In traditional Chinese medicine, concepts such as consciousness, feeling and thought are referred to as *shen*, meaning 'mind' (although often translated as 'spirit'). The *shen* governs all physiological functions of the major organs (heart, liver, lung, spleen and kidney). There are seven emotions, or *qī qíng*, which when experienced in excess (compared to normal everyday reactions to common events) can cause dis-*ease*. The spleen is the organ correlated with anxiety, and the Chinese herbs prescribed to treat the spleen cleared up the phlegm that was causing my asthma—and my anxiety evaporated.

Yet I still hadn't learned how to identify my emotions or express my feelings. Seven or so years later, when Steve was diagnosed with cancer just before I turned 40, I was completely ill-equipped to deal with the realities of his terminal illness and to accept he was dying. After beating myself up for quite a long time, I came to appreciate that growing up in a WEIRD (Western, educated, industrialised, rich and democratic) culture was partly why I hadn't developed the skills to support him, or myself.

Canadian author Stephen Jenkinson believes the North American culture is 'death phobic'. In *Die Wise: A Manifesto for Sanity and Soul*, he asks how natural it is to be afraid of dying.

> If it is natural, that should mean that everyone—or everyone who is following their nature, or everyone who is sane—should be more or less afraid to die, or prone to it. It should mean that being human and being alive means being afraid to die.

Yet, as he goes on to argue, infants don't seem to show any fear. Children are afraid of strangers because we tell them to be. They are afraid of falling down stairs if they have done it before. But they don't seem to be afraid of dying. Instead, he suggests, we have to *learn* to be afraid to die.

Psychotherapists might suggest that attachment theories account for my anxiety. They might suggest that the routines and rituals I've adopted could be described as obsessive-compulsive disorder. But I don't care much for labels. They can, in many ways, confine one to a particular behaviour paradigm. I also question the focus on individual personality traits, when often it's the way our society and culture works that can have the most impact. We need to examine sociology as much as psychology.

Jenkinson also interrogates the link between fear of death and attachment theories:

> Writers who are fond of 'attachment theories' as the bases for a healthy emotional life argue that close relationships teach that kind of anxiety, that having breeds the fear of losing. The greater exposure people have to dying, which the psychological literature calls loss, and the more they have to lose, the more they have to fear.[3]

---

3 *Die Wise* (Berkeley, CA: North Atlantic Books, 2015), Chapter 5, Kindle.

As he points out, the opposite often appears to be true. We in the WEIRD world, certainly since the late 60s, when I was born, have much less exposure to dying people and corpses. There is far less dying for people to see. Most dying takes place in hospitals, and the majority of us pay funeral directors to prepare our loved ones' bodies for burial or cremation.

'The pervasive fear of dying in the adult population ... doesn't come from seeing more dying as people get older,' Jenkinson concludes. 'It comes, partly, from seeing not much dying or much death at all as they get older.'[4]

Before Steve died, I certainly didn't have many, or any, opportunities to express my fears that those I loved *might* die. Even when he was diagnosed with cancer, we refused to utter the D word. It was as if I believed that acknowledging the possibility of death would make it happen. As if even thinking he might die would make it so. As if my inner thoughts determined his fate.

How strange, when of course it should be 'those I loved *would* die'. Not necessarily today or tomorrow, but for as long as I'm still breathing, people I love *will* die.

No one could have prepared me for the fact that being with my first husband when he died did not make me fear death more, but less. Then, as I struggled to adapt to life without him, the anxiety returned. Yet it was new blend of anxiety, a realisation after his death that control over anything, bar our thoughts, is an illusion.

I have been fortunate: I am not isolated. I am part of a supportive community and have developed enduring personal relationships with others; I can step out my front door and be amongst nature; my days are filled with meaningful endeavours. These are all precursors for good mental health. Assuming this foundation for a connected and meaningful life exists, I've discovered three steps that help me manage anxiety. The first

---

4   Ibid.

step is to identify and acknowledge my feelings and emotions. The second, to learn how to express them. The third and most important step seems the simplest of all, but in my experience has often been the most difficult: to shut up and focus on my breath.

On the eve of David's departure on the three passes tramp, we stopped for lunch in Hokitika. Our friend Chaitanya Deva, a Nelson-based massage therapist and yoga teacher, was a member of the tramping party.

As we ate, he told me how he has noticed, after decades of practising and teaching meditation, that people exhibiting anxious behaviours tend to hold their breath after breathing in, delaying the exhalation. In contrast those in a depressive state hold their breath after breathing out, delaying the inhalation.

This was a revelation for me. Of course, that's exactly what I do: I forget to breathe out. Bringing my awareness to the exhalation is like pushing a reset button. I stop filling myself up with oxygen like the goldfish in the toilet bowl and start breathing in a natural rhythm again.

Now, during nocturnal visits from anxiety, I focus not only on my breath in an unspecified way, but on the exhalation itself. And I remember this mantra: *Death is always coming. Right now, I'm alive. Breathe.* It's a meditation. As Dispenza says, meditation means 'become familiar with'.[5]

According to the philosopher Spinoza, a *free person* is not anxious about death. In other words, contemplating death, and making peace with death, can be profoundly liberating.

---

5   Dispenza, *Breaking the Habit of Being Yourself* (Hay House, 2012), 176.

Anxiety in the Body

Rosemary Mannering

When Jane came into my clinic, she walked stiffly. She sat in the chair closest to the door, her eyes flitting around the room as she assessed any possible threats, twisting and wringing the strap of her handbag. I thought I could slide a sheet of newspaper between her and the seat of the chair. Jane had come to my specialist physiotherapy service to learn to recognise and to control her anxiety through muscle relaxation and correct breathing patterns.

In 1982 my family and I moved back to Christchurch from where I had been working as a physiotherapist in a rural community and hospital. I spoke to the director of physiotherapy services at the North Canterbury Hospital Board and enquired after a position. As I remember, she asked if I would be 'prepared to go out to Sunnyside'—the local psychiatric hospital. My heart raced, my hands sweated and my mind shut down. I squeaked a yes. I was assured that, after four months, there would be a vacancy for me at the general hospital. With great fear and total ignorance, I went out to Sunnyside to treat patients who were extremely psychiatrically ill.

In spite of my initial reluctance, I found a sense of reward in helping psychiatrically ill patients through physiotherapy. I stayed at Sunnyside Hospital for 20 years before establishing my specialist physiotherapy clinic, where I continue to teach individuals to calm their anxiety by relaxing muscle tension and breathing diaphragmatically.

Jane had come to my clinic to learn to control her anxiety. When she came in that first day, she was in fight or flight mode, ready to run from the room or hit out to defend herself. And yet, she was sitting in a chair—so all her physical tension and rapid breathing was unnecessary. The disparity between how she felt and what she was doing physically meant she was experiencing a dry mouth, nausea, a racing heart, shortness of breath, and shaking and tingling sensations in her hands and feet.

Jane's counsellor had sent me a letter in advance of her appointment. Jane, she explained, was a conscientious mother of two children, eleven and nine years old. At the time of the Christchurch earthquake, the children had been taken from their central city school to the botanic gardens as a place of safety. Jane, meanwhile, was at home during the earthquake when the chimney crashed through the roof of the lounge. She was unhurt but frightened. As her cellphone was buried in the rubble, she lost her main method of contact with her children. Always an anxious person, the effect of this on Jane was catastrophic. It was two agonising hours before she found where her children were being cared for. Since then, the counsellor wrote to me, Jane has suffered from flashbacks and nightmares, reliving different aspects of that afternoon and her panic of not knowing where her children were and if they were safe. Post-traumatic stress disorder, the counsellor wrote.

After giving Jane time to be comfortable with me and reassuring her by asking simple questions, the wringing of her handbag strap slowed and her hands became less tense. Eventually, I asked her if she was conscious of all the muscles she was holding so tightly. Jane was aware of muscle fatigue and pain, but not of the tightness she was exhibiting. Jane had been holding her muscles tighter than necessary to do daily activities—they were tight enough to climb Mount Cook, I told her! No wonder she was sore all the time.

'Freeze,' I said. 'Don't move anywhere and see if you can feel any muscles working.' Jane's posture didn't change as she focussed on her body sensations for a moment. 'What can you feel?' I asked. Jane found it hard to answer. Recognising muscle tension when it is so habitual is difficult. Jane's instructions were to 'freeze' and be still, 'feel' by recognising muscle tension, 'flop' by actively letting all unnecessary muscles stop working and then to 'feel the difference'. The idea was that, with practice, Jane would become more aware of her habitual patterns of body tension and learn to reduce them.

As Jane began to recognise where her body held muscles tightly, she learned to focus on specific areas and to relax the muscles there. Together, we grouped them into six areas: shoulders, hands, abdomen, buttocks, feet and mouth.

Firstly, we addressed the shoulders. Jane realised that she held her shoulders up towards her ears. There may be some biological reasoning for this, giving the appearance of power and aggression, but we don't need to hold up our shoulders unless we are being physically active. Hesitantly, Jane lowered her shoulders, feeling that as she did so the tension in her neck and across her shoulder girdle eased. Initially, she found this sensation odd.

Next, we talked about Jane's hand-wringing actions and the handbag strap that had been bent and twisted like overworked putty. It took courage for Jane to put the handbag out of reach and to let her hands rest without being clenched into fists.

Then Jane discovered that, as she sat forward in the chair, she was holding her abdominal muscles tightly. She recognised that she had always tried to hold her stomach in—partly because she thought she looked better with her stomach held in, but also it kept her in a braced posture. When Jane dropped her shoulders, relaxed her abdominal muscles and let her hands rest on her lap, she admitted she felt calmer.

We discussed the tension in her buttock and thigh muscles. The buttock muscles work to move our hip joints into a straight position, and when sitting they should be relaxed and lengthened. Jane's muscles had not relaxed; they had only stretched enough to bend her hips as far as was essential for her to sit, and were ready to tighten more at any moment, to lift her into a standing position. After several appointments, Jane learned to reduce the tightness in her buttocks. 'Sit on soft, squidgy cushions,' I told her, 'not hard knobbly ones.' Jane noticed that when she let her buttock muscles relax, her knees shifted apart a little, to a position equal to the width of her shoulders.

Paddling her feet up and down and curling her toes were habitual actions of Jane's. Once she was able to relax her buttock muscles, she found letting her feet be heavy on the floor became a more natural feeling.

Finally, we addressed her mouth. Everyone clenches their teeth together at times of pressure, bracing the teeth in the lower jaw against the top teeth. This protective action prevents the teeth from being damaged if they should come together suddenly—say, if a person falls and their jaw hits a hard surface. It is a powerful reflex, used but unnecessary, when the threat of danger is perceived but not physical. The muscles used to bring the jaw tightly closed can be felt in the cheeks and the temples. Jane could feel these muscles working as she put her hands and fingers against her cheeks and temples and alternately clenched and relaxed her jaw. I asked Jane to clench her jaw and notice the action of her tongue. She was surprised to discover it became firm and tight. Then, when encouraged to relax her tongue, her teeth released their pressure and her jaw dropped slightly. When Jane's tongue was soft in her mouth, it rested gently on the roof of her mouth.

Relaxing the tension in Jane's tongue became the focus of her body relaxation. When we speak, our tongue moves, allowing us to make different sounds. Jane found that when she said the letter 'n', even in her head rather than aloud, her tongue would gently dock on the roof of her mouth and her jaw tension would relax. Furthermore, when her tongue relaxed, her shoulders would drop further and her abdominal muscles would loosen. Jane now uses a word ending in 'n' as a distraction and mantra when she's feeling panicked. That helps relax her whole body.

After recognising her habitual muscle tension and developing skills to reduce it, Jane learnt to recognise her breathing pattern. I told Jane that when her shoulders are elevated and her abdominal muscles are held tightly, her breathing pattern is affected, causing all the movement to occur in her upper chest. As she sat back in her chair with her knees shoulder-width apart and her shoulders down, Jane became aware that her breathing rate had slowed and, for the first time in years, she could see her stomach gently swelling as she breathed in and gently sinking as she breathed out. Exploring the movement, when she leaned forward, her breathing moved further up into her chest. Similarly, when she held her knees together and raised her shoulders, the abdominal movement when breathing was reduced and breaths became shorter.

By recognising and reducing muscle tension, Jane learnt that she could correct the breathing pattern that occurs when she is anxious and that can lead to panic attacks. I explained that the major muscle for breathing is the diaphragm, which lies across the lower chest, beneath the lungs. As it contracts, it moves downwards and displaces the abdominal contents slightly, causing the stomach to swell. When the diaphragm relaxes it moves up again, allowing the stomach to sink in and the air to flow out of the lungs in a relaxed expiration. Jane practised this movement lying down. She liked the feeling of the gentle abdominal movement. She checked for areas of muscle tension. Were her shoulders down? Were her knees a little apart? Was her head heavy against the pillow? Was her tongue relaxed? Once she was sure she had relaxed all the muscle groups she was aware of, she focussed on the sensation of her stomach rising and sinking as she breathed in and out.

Breathing should always be a gentle and comfortable activity. Air flows into the lungs as the diaphragm moves downwards, stretching the lungs and creating vacuum. Then the diaphragm moves up as it stops working; the wondrously elastic lungs shrink and the air flows out. Jane felt a tiny pause before she breathed in again. Just for a moment, the action of breathing rested before the next breath, in and straight out, and then a momentary pause—'in, out, pause; in, out, pause'. She learnt that airflow should be both in and out through the nose. When anxiety influences muscle tension and breathing patterns, the moment of pause is lost and more rapid or irregular breathing occurs, often through the mouth.

Anxiety attacks are associated with hyperventilation, which occurs when breathing is out of proportion to the amount of physical activity at the time. I explained to Jane that, when she is anxious and is breathing rapidly, she has sufficient oxygen at all times but feels short of breath because she is breathing out too much of the carbon dioxide that her body is making. The reduction of carbon dioxide in her blood upsets the normal balance of oxygen and carbon dioxide, causing the many physical symptoms she experiences—hyperventilation syndrome.

Prolonging the pause between breaths can correct this physiological imbalance. Following the 'in, out, pause' pattern deliberately slows the breathing, and that momentary delay before breathing in allows the level of carbon dioxide to increase. As Jane learned to breathe diaphragmatically at a rate of approximately 12 breaths per minute, she found she was able to reduce the many physical symptoms of her anxiety. When in situations which caused her anxiety to increase, she learnt to actively drop her shoulders and consciously slow her breathing rate by delaying before each breath in. Jane now carries a small card around in her wallet, on which is written:

First Aid for Panic
Drop your shoulders

Breathe in, breathe out
Delay before you breathe in
Remember *nnnnn*.

After several months of increasingly widely spaced appointments, I discharged Jane from treatment. She had learned to recognise when she was tensing her muscles and to reduce tightness by actively relaxing her muscle tension, sitting in a comfortable position in a chair and breathing in a calm, regulated diaphragmatic pattern. We laughed as we recalled her robotic figure from day one, who had sat seemingly above—not on—the chair. Jane still remembers the day of the earthquake, but she no longer has PTSD. At the time of discharge, she had not had a panic attack for several months.

Earnest PSA

Susan Strongman

She is putting her coat and bag in the back room at Golden Dawn, like she always does when it's busy and hot and she wants to dance. She's come to the bar with friends. They want to dance too.

The room is tiny and dark and humid, almost an alcove. A thick wool curtain separates it from the rest of the bar. As she pushes it aside, it falls behind her and the music is muffled. For a moment she lingers in the warmth and darkness.

Then she hears the curtain jerked open behind her. The music is loud again and a woman is shouting, *You can't be here! Get out! Who are you! What are you doing!*

Her heart starts to race. She tries to explain, but all she can hear is the woman shouting. Her heart is pounding, throbbing inside her chest but also inside her skull and all of her body. The music is sharp and loud and she tries to explain that she's allowed to put her coat here and she does it all the time and this bar is a safe bar, her friend's bar, but the shouting woman is not listening.

She backs away, further into the tiny room, her hands prickling. She's drowning. The room is a black hole. It's hard to breathe. She can't breathe.

She runs out of the room like a scared cat, and there are her friends. But it's too loud and bright out here. Faces are staring at her, puzzled, and she is trying to tell her friends what's happening, but are they her friends? Why is she crying? Don't make a scene.

The panic won't stop, and she needs to go.

Someone is following her, and then he is holding her arm,

tugging. *Come back! Don't be a dick!*
Go away! She's shouting now too. *Leave me alone! I'm going home!* She is running and he is following.

Headlights, red man, car horns. He is still following her. She shoves him. Twice. She yells. She swears. She sobs and runs.

At home she calls a friend, but it's late and her friend hangs up. She calls again. He hangs up. Again she calls him. His phone is turned off now. She leaves frantic messages. She is not calm.

Her cat is in her bedroom. Sweet little grey cat with one eye. Juno will calm her. But she is sobbing, and Juno is scared of her; her eye is wide and fearful. *Why are you doing this?* Juno's eye is saying. She scampers under the bed.

She sobs harder. Her flatmates will hear but she doesn't care. She turns out the light and gets into bed and pulls the heavy duvet over. Blackness. Face-down on her pillow, her sobs and gasps for air are muffled. Snot and drool and tears and the mascara and orange lipstick from this night will never wash out of her pillowcase.

In the morning, the thought of it brings the tingling back. She made a scene last night. Her head aches from booze and tears and she has the fear and she will be tired for days.

A friend tells her it's okay. You just had a blow-out, she says. The friend is kind. She cooks soft boiled eggs with soldiers and they go for a walk and pet horses and later they light a fire at the friend's nice house, and curl up in blankets and watch movies and the friend doesn't ask what happened, but the friend is there and the friend listens.

But she is still worried—paranoid, maybe. People talk; they laugh at her. She's the girl who cried at the bar. They call her crazy. Nuts. Emotional. Sometimes they react with anger. She has been like this forever so she's used to it, but she hates it still. Until she was in her late 20s, she'd just thought she was angry and mental, defective. She didn't have a name for panic attacks.

She wants her friends to understand that she doesn't want to be like this, and that she tries so hard not to let it happen—the panic, tears and anger. She tries to avoid unfamiliar social situations. Avoid bad people. Don't get too tired. Sneak home before you make a scene. Don't let it escalate. Find a quiet place and be calm. Breathe. Count. Feel your muscles relax. Take a pill if you must.

Amid her anger, she tells herself that it's not her fault when other people don't try to understand. She can choose who to spend her time with. If they laugh at you, they are not your friends. If they tell the funny story about the girl who cried at the bar, they are not your friends. If they are angry at you and are sick of your shit, they are not your friends. If they take offence because they misunderstood, they are not your friends. Tell their mates to avoid her. She's crazy. Take your pills. Don't take your pills. Read this self-help book. Call her emotional. Put *Manic Depression* on a mixtape and give it to her for Christmas.

She has very few friends.

Back home with her cats, she opens Facebook. *What's on your mind?*

I have a mental illness—depression, which comes with a generous side of anxiety.

I have panic attacks. There are some things that set me off, and sometimes I just have them for no reason. When I have a panic attack my heart races. Then I cry.

This has been happening since I was a teen, and my closest friends know all about it. Some are still my friends, others aren't. It's not easy being friends with depression and anxiety. Especially if you don't understand it.

Does she want sympathy? Support? Attention? Does she worry if she speaks about it to real friends she will burden them with her madness? Did she write the post so the friends at the bar would see it? Did she want them to see it because she was angry at them? Did she want them to see how they'd made her feel as they stared at her, baffled, as tears rolled down her cheeks, or as they told her not to be a dick when she'd wanted to go home, or when they'd laughed about it among themselves the following day?

Is the post manipulative? Neurotic? Is she writing it because she wants people to know she's not crazy, she's just sick; that anxiety made her panic? That she's not really like that?

She wants to tell people that it's not okay to laugh at her anxiety. It's not okay to call her nuts or emotional or tell her to take drugs or not to take drugs. Yes, she has a good doctor. No, she can't afford this psychologist. Thank you for the tip about mindfulness and meditation. *Thank you for the link to the self-help book—I will check it out!* She won't.

She writes that she knows you were laughing about her because you didn't know how to react. But did you know that in doing so, you were laughing at mental illness?

I want people to be aware that mental illness is a thing that people, fucking heaps of people, have to deal with and someone having a meltdown shouldn't be something you tell your mates about because you think it's funny.

She writes that she would like people to be more tolerant and understanding. Kind, even, like her friend was, the morning after, with the soft boiled eggs and the horses.

She agonises over the settings on the post. Her Facebook connections are a ragtag group of school friends, former colleagues, people she has met on overseas holidays and friends of friends of friends. She is opening up about her mental illness. She knows people will judge her for it, people who don't know her. Who will she allow to see that she's weak and mad?

But then she doesn't care anymore, and she hits the post button and closes Facebook and forgets about it.

She can't remember what she does in the hours after her

post goes up. She probably sleeps. After a panic attack, she feels weak for days. Tired and empty, like she's got the flu.

Later, the anxiety sets in again. She doesn't want to check Facebook. Why did she post that? It doesn't fit with her self-presentation. They'll know she's neurotic. *You just want attention*, she imagines them saying. *Or acceptance! Revenge!*

208 likes. 60 comments. Two dozen messages. Jesus Christ, what have you done?

I'm glad this post popped up in my timeline. Cos I would be more alone without it.

I have had a mental illness and I am thankful for your announcement.

Thanks for the candour.

Every time someone is honest about living with mental illness it makes it easier for the rest of us.

Sorry you had such a shit time and I hope you're having some better days. You're a brave and strong woman.

No one has called her nuts or emotional or left a laughing face emoji on the post. The person who chased her doesn't see it, because she has unfriended him on Facebook and in real life too.

A friend tells another friend that he saw the post and thinks it's about him. The friend is annoyed that she posted it on social media rather than talking to him about it in person. She tells the friend to reign in his ego; the post was not about him.

She changes the post settings to private so that no one but her can see it ever again. She no longer trusts her friends from that night. She's still ashamed; she still feels defective. After all, that's what anxiety is, right? A defect? Something that a person should hide from the people around them?

But she knows that the post and the nice comments are there. Every now and then, she goes back to it, to read the good things that people have written.

Side Effects

Paula Harris

It was Friday the 13th. That isn't a joke; it isn't some literary device to further this piece. It actually was Friday the 13th. I had a meeting at 9:30a.m. with my new hospital psychiatrist. People said to me beforehand that Friday the 13th is awesome, that this was a good sign and that this meeting—my fourth psychiatrist in six months—would go well. It's Friday the 13th! It'll be great!

Spoiler alert: It wasn't great.

I'd had a really rough week. My hospital psychologist was away for the school holidays, so I hadn't seen him for a fortnight. I was sad and hope-lost and so very sick of myself, because that's what severe depression is like. I had been due to meet with my Community Mental Health Services key worker, Jimmy, on the Wednesday. (A key worker is your primary contact at CMHS, there to help you navigate essential services.) This was a stop-gap measure to talk with someone while my psychologist was away, but, at the last minute, Jimmy had to cancel when another of his patients had a crisis.

I was anxious about having to meet with the new psychiatrist, because the last one had made me really uncomfortable; I'd walked out within 90 seconds of him commanding me to sit down. Because the new psychiatrist was going to be the 13th mental health professional I'd seen, which meant I'd have to explain all my background stuff for the 13th time, and I'm so exhausted by having to talk new people through all of this. Because at some point he'd ask me if I think about suicide and I'd say yes, and he'd ask me if I had a plan and I'd say yes, and he'd ask me to tell him my plan and I'd say no, and he'd frown and push me for details, because that's the interaction I'd had so many times before. Because I was anxious about sleeping through my alarm, because my depression is exhausting and I struggle to wake up.

I'd never thought of myself as someone who had anxiety. I tend to be shy and introverted, so I can feel stressed when having to deal with strangers, especially in large groups, but at the same time I'm used to teaching groups of people—in my life I've taught Pilates and massage and Italian cooking and Argentine tango—and being loud and funny and outgoing, and that being a part of who I am. As my current episode of depression has progressed—as I write this, we're nearly three years into this episode—I have retreated more and more from the world, so that when I do have to go out and interact with people, I get stressed and, yes, I become anxious. My psychologist, the Lovely Harry (his name is Harry and he's quite lovely), told me that this is called social anxiety. My social anxiety really only became real, as opposed to me feeling stressed around people, as a result of one of the antidepressants I was taking. I can't even remember which one it was now—there have been so many antidepressants—but I remember how it gave me chest-crushing palpitations. And somewhere along the line, while my ribs felt strapped down by the medication and my heart was trying to escape, somewhere in the middle of that, social anxiety found a spot to plant itself. In the fertile manure of my depression, it grew well.

On Friday the 13th I *was* five minutes late to my psychiatrist appointment. I *had* overslept a little—why do hospitals make psychiatric appointments for the morning, when a sizeable number of psych patients struggle in the morning?—and had rushed to have a shower and eat breakfast and get dressed and walk the seven minutes from my house to the hospital. Community Mental Health Services is the home for psych outpatient treatment. It's housed in an old two-storey brick building that would be stunning if someone showed it some care.

Jimmy came to get me from the waiting room, because your key worker sits in on your psychiatrist appointments. The mental health system has fucked me around since I was referred into it by my GP, and I tend to push back when I feel that people are messing me around, so Jimmy is my third key worker. I like Jimmy. My patient file at CMHS notes my trust issues with people, including (possibly especially) with CMHS staff. The Lovely Harry had told me, before he left for his holiday, that I need to take chances; I need to give people the opportunity to not disappoint or hurt me.

I won't refer to my psychiatrist by his real name. The simple fact is that hearing or saying his name triggers an anxiety attack. And I don't need that shit. I call him Voldemort instead.

Voldemort didn't give me bad vibes straight away, not like my third psychiatrist had. But, whereas numbers one and two had been open and engaging in their energy, he was aloof and closed off. My inclination was not to answer his questions, but I kept thinking about Harry telling me to take chances and trust someone. I kept thinking about how I needed to be upfront with people so that they could help me get better. I was depressed and worn out, and then Voldemort asked, 'Do you think about suicide?'

I told him, 'Yes.'
'Do you have a plan?'
I slipped deeper into my chair. 'Yes.'
'Can you tell me your plan?'
'No.'

Everything in the room changed. It was as if someone had mixed cornflour into the air to make it thicker. Voldemort's body tensed, as if every cell inside him had shrunk.

Because you'll ask, I don't tell anyone my plan. Because it's the security blanket I curl into when I'm having a really bad day, knowing that there is a way out. Because I don't want to risk anyone taking that from me.

The long story involves two hours of papers being shuffled and people talking about me in hallways and Voldemort and another psychiatrist—who met me for all of five minutes—signing paperwork. The long story involves my realisation that as soon as I said *yes*, no one would listen to anything I said after that. The long story feels surreal. The long story is about how it felt like all of this was a joke, a misunderstanding, and any second now it would all be cleared up.

The short story is that I was admitted, under the Mental Health (Compulsory Assessment and Treatment) Act 1992, to the secure unit of the psychiatric ward just after noon on Friday the 13th.

Being sectioned has various time frames. Your sectioning can be cancelled early, if an appropriately authorised person signs a form to say that you are no longer mentally unsound, but otherwise the first time frame is five days. At the end of the five days, if you are not released, there is a further 14 days. After the 14 days, the time frame moves forward in periods of six months.

'We've just finished making up your room,' I was told, as if I was staying in a nice hotel. My cell consisted of an upholstered plinth and a mattress, along with a pillow and sheets, which I was repeatedly reminded that I should be grateful to have been allowed. I sat down on my mattress. I was shock and confused and alone. I had no real idea as to how things had reached this point. I realised that whatever I had done wrong that got me declared mentally unsound on day one wasn't going to go away by day five. And then I'd be here for another 14 days. And I didn't know what I could say on day 19 that would change things, so then I'd be here for six months.

That is when I truly developed anxiety.

The ward staff rang my emergency contact, and I was shown to the phone booth to talk with her. Her only concern was how she could get me sufficient supplies of clean underwear. How could she get into my house? Was there a spare key somewhere? She could go to Farmers and buy me some, if that would work? Did someone else have a spare key to my house?

All I wanted to do was cry. I couldn't see how I was ever going to get out.

I was tired and scared and alone and hungry. The ward staff had promised to bring me some lunch when they finished admitting me, but they forgot until sometime after four o'clock. They gave me a plate of ham sandwiches, even though I'd said that I don't eat pork products. They sighed. I pulled the bread away from the ham and ate that, and then found one egg sandwich at the bottom of the stack.

I pushed back at the psych ward system. I wanted to see a psychiatrist. Surely, if I saw someone other than Voldemort, they'd realise that this was all some crazy mix-up and would let me out. Or, at least, they would start me on a new antidepressant, since that had been my main aim for my appointment with Voldemort. The nurses kept telling me I wouldn't be released 'until you get better', and, to me, starting medication seemed like the best way for me to start getting better. The ward psychiatrist—whom I'd initially been told I'd see on Friday afternoon—had finished for the week, but I found out that there was an on-call psych registrar. I asked for them to be paged. I was told they could only be paged if there was a reason. I stared down the nurse and said, 'It's my right as a patient to see a doctor.' She frowned at me, and left.

The psych registrar showed up around ten at night. He made it very clear from the start that he had no interest in taking any active steps. He wouldn't prescribe me any medication. He wouldn't tell me what I needed to do 'to get better'. I'd have to wait until the ward psychiatrist arrived on Monday before anyone would discuss medications or treatment with me. I would spend three days of my initial five-day time frame without any form of treatment, but I'd only get out on day five if I was better. It seemed impossible.

I was tired and scared and alone and I tried to go to sleep. In the secure cells the light switches are flat metal buttons. I closed the blind, which was secure between two panes of glass, and pressed the buttons so that I could have darkness. But only one light went out. I pressed the buttons again. Still, light. I tried the button on the other side of the room. Still, light. I pressed the button to page a nurse.

When the nurse arrived she told me, 'You have to have the light on. You're *at risk*.'

'But the light's right over me. I can't sleep with the light in my face.'

'You can have the light turned off once you get better.'

I lay on my bed thinking about how I was never going to get out, because I can't sleep if it isn't dark and therefore I was never going to get better. At some point the nurse came back and showed me where the main light control was for my room so that I would stop crying.

Finally, I had darkness. I cried quieter. The nurse shone her torch through my window every ten minutes.

I didn't like how quickly I got used to the rhythms of the secure unit. There are just six beds, six cells; a maximum of six patients.

One nurse for every two patients. My morning nurse came in to wake me up and was surprised by my irritability.

'I spent all night cold and tired and hungry,' I said, 'why the fuck would I be irritable?'

The afternoon nurse brought me a blanket and told me that they could, technically, order me snacks from the hospital kitchen.

The night nurse tut-tutted that I had been given a blanket, since I was *at risk* and therefore should have nothing.

By Saturday lunchtime I was the only female patient in the unit. I was 20 years older than any of the others. I kept to myself, staying in my cell unless I had visitors and was in the interview room. I swung between freaking out that I was in the psych ward and accepting that I would be there forever. How can you possibly get out when you don't know how you got there?

At this point my medical notes start to comment that I was improving. But I was giving up.

On the Monday I was woken by a nurse, as the ward psychiatrist was waiting to see me. I didn't know what to expect. I was tired and scared and alone. I didn't want to say the wrong thing again. I didn't know the right thing to say. My head was still bogged down inside the little sleep I'd managed in those last few hours of night. I went into my bathroom, where I could tuck myself behind the door to get dressed out of view. The nurse was irritated that I was taking too long and called from the door to see if I was going to meet with the psychiatrist. 'I'm just fucking getting dressed!' I yelled back at her. I finished putting on my socks—you can tell the patients from the staff because patients shuffle around in socks, our shoes taken from us due to the laces—and scuttled across to the interview room.

The ward psychiatrist had a thick American accent. Her energy wasn't tightly wired like Voldemort's had been; she was relaxed and alert on the couch. I slouched into the chair opposite my nurse and a registrar, who wrote notes throughout. I didn't know what the right things to say were and was too tired to filter my words. She asked what had happened that had gotten me admitted to the ward; I told her that my psychiatrist was a dickhead. But then we talked. She was yet another mental health professional whom I had to explain my stuff to.

'Well,' she said in that way only Americans can say *well*, 'there are two types of suicidality—acute and chronic.' She felt that I was in the category of chronic, and in those cases treatment is best out in the community rather than in the psych ward. She was comfortable with the idea of discharging me, if Harry agreed. I would be transferred to the open side of the psych ward, to start 'transitioning' back to the outside world.

I remember snorting inside that I would need to 'transition'. She said I might be released! Bring on the outside world!

My nurse took me for a tour of the open side of the ward. After the smaller, darker space of the secure unit, suddenly there was so much stimulation. I was overwhelmed by the people, the light, the voices. I stuck close to the nurse and shuffled back to the secure unit behind her. It took a couple of hours before a room was ready for me in the open side, and I didn't want to go. I knew the secure unit, I felt safe there—and I felt freaked out at feeling safe there. But they needed my cell for someone else.

My new room had a window that could open, and shelves and light switches and two chairs and an actual hospital bed. I stayed in my room. A visitor arrived for me, and we went into one of the interview rooms, where we could lock ourselves in and not be disturbed by anyone. The furniture was awkward but I fell asleep on a beanbag, my visitor stroking my arm as I slept.

I was released just before five o'clock. Harry had told the ward psychiatrist that he thought it was the worst place I could be. My visitor stuck around until all the paperwork was finished and I was given the letter officially declaring me to be mentally sound. There was a brief joy of walking out of the ward and to her car, so that she could drive me and my accumulated belongings—poetry books, pens, notebooks, underwear—back home.

But once I was home, I struggled to return to the outside world. The next day, Tuesday, I had a scheduled appointment with Harry. The seven-minute walk took closer to 15, as I had to stop for an anxiety attack along the way. When I arrived, Harry led me through to the room where we have our sessions, and I cried and hyperventilated.

Over the next two months I spent so much time rubbing the tight spot on my sternum, just trying to breathe, that I was amazed I didn't bruise. Harry encouraged me to take long exhales. I felt as though an alien would burst out of my chest.

My fear of being put back in the psych ward is a travelling storm that hovers above me. Harry reassures me that it won't happen, that I won't go back, that the ward psychiatrist would most likely refuse Voldemort if he tried to admit me again, but the rational argument doesn't convince the reflex fear to go away. And every week I have to walk with that anxiety to CMHS. To walk into the building that Voldemort is in. To know that people can choose *not* to hear me and force me into hospital against my will, a power no other medical speciality has. To fear saying something wrong and being readmitted.

Anxiety is the gift that my fourth psychiatrist, and the psych ward, gave me.

I don't leave the house much anymore. The anxiety became so overwhelming that, whenever I tried to work, I would spend the first five minutes of every Pilates session crying and struggling to breathe in the corner. Getting there had exhausted me and now there were all these people—my warm, loving clients—who I had to think about. I hated that I was doing this to my clients, so I closed my business of 20 years.

I have strategies to help me get to my weekly session with Harry. I never have an appointment earlier than eleven o'clock, so that I won't get too anxious about oversleeping. When I wake up, and again before I leave the house, I use an essential oil blend to help calm me, putting a small amount at the base of my skull and on my sternum, where the alien wants to break through. I use a homeopathic spray to help calm me down as I sit in the waiting room.

For the first couple of months after being sectioned, I wore clothes that I felt I could run away in. Now I try to wear things that make me feel good. I put on my headphones and listen to music while I walk to my appointment. Aretha Franklin's 'Think' is particularly effective while crossing the hospital carpark. *It don't take too much high IQs / To see what you're doing to me . . .*

If it's a really rough day, I'll keep my headphones on while I sit in the waiting room. If I can stay inside the music, then the anxiety has less space to grab hold of.

Harry helps by trying to book us into the same meeting room each week, so that I'll be in a familiar environment. Every week he tells me to do whatever I need to in order make the room more comfortable, to open or close the windows, to shift the chairs around. What I really want is for the room to not be in the same building as Voldemort. To not be in the same building as Community Mental Health Services.

Voldemort's decision made me stop trusting myself. He took away my power when I was incredibly vulnerable.

I want to not feel anxiety sprinting through my body anytime my heart rate goes up a little. I want to not feel that air is repelled by my body. I want to not have nightmares every single night. I want to talk openly with Harry and not hold back because I'm terrified that this might be the thing that changes his mind and makes him call out for a psychiatrist. I want to walk up my street without feeling anxious because I'm walking vaguely in the direction of the hospital. I want to not cry when I get mail from CMHS. I want to not jump whenever the phone rings, because I think they—the hospital, the police—are on their way to take me back in.

I want to go back to the old me, the person who just got hung up about having to meet new people. The me who was still here on Thursday the 12th.

Writing from a Dark Place

Lee Murray

When I was six years old, I imagined there was a wolf under my bed.

Dad insisted there was nothing there. 'There *are* no wolves in New Zealand,' he said, 'and there are none under your bed.' He lifted the bedspread. 'See?'

But I could hear it, prowling and pacing on the floor beneath me. I tried to block the sound, burying my ear against the pillow, but it was still there, a lone male with yellow gleaming eyes and blood-blackened teeth.

That wolf has been visiting me for a long time now. Keeping me awake, worrying at me.

Sometimes, he sits on my chest in the darkness until I can't breathe. Even though I've known for years that the sound of those paws is nothing more than my own pulse thrumming in my ear.

And there are no wolves in New Zealand.

'Of course, you're a worrier,' explains my Chinese mother. She's referring to the little dark mole on my back near my left shoulder. Moles on the back are always a bad omen. A mole on the shoulder means you're burdened with the world's troubles. My birthdate doesn't help: in the Chinese zodiac, I'm a wood snake. Snakes are known to be great thinkers. They hate to fail, and they stress out a lot. Even my Chinese name, Wei-Hahn, can mean perfection, which is easy enough to achieve when you're a tiny baby, but keeping that up your whole life? It's as if the gods have set me up, as if I was destined to be a worrier from the get-go.

The official diagnoses of anxiety and depression from

my doctor came much later, almost five decades. The news surprised me at first, as it does a lot of people when I tell them—although, admittedly, I haven't told many.

'Anxiety? You? But you're so happy and bubbly.'

'Really? You're always so positive. So *smiley*.'

And outwardly I am.

It's just inwardly that I tend to overthink things. Ruminate on them. Obsess. I spend hours pondering people's responses and composing better answers in my head. Wondering what I might have done, or not done, to offend them. My mind races and my stomach sours. My muscles tense and cramp. I stay up late and don't sleep much.

Sometimes, going out is too hard, so I make an excuse and stay home. Or staying out is too hard, so I duck out early and go home.

Let's back up a bit. Late nights. No sleep. Obsessing over every word. A tendency towards introversion. Taken together, don't those habits sound a lot like a writer?

Think about it: writers are scholars of human behaviour. Our entire lives are subject to study: every interaction carved up and examined, the way a scientist might examine a cadaver, and then we record those observations in our writing. If you're a horror writer like me, you might even introduce a few cadavers to the plot, raising the stakes to create the worse-case scenario, just to see how the protagonist responds. And then, when we have captured the essence of the story, we go back and scrutinise every sentence. Revise, edit, rewrite. Repeat. Polishing and perfecting the words. Overthinking on paper.

Sometimes, sending the work out is too hard; we can't bear to face criticism, so we keep it at home in a folder. Or, if we do send it out, the wait will be interminable.

And, assuming we aren't ghosted by a publisher or an agent, when the long-anticipated mail does come in, we pore over the rejection, trying to work out what we might have done wrong. Could I have phrased that better, maybe chosen a better angle? Did I misread the submission guidelines? Even when the work is published and paid for, we worry that no one will read it. Or if they do, will they like it?

It's as if anxiety and writing are synonymous.

Hardly surprising then that creative, successful people are eight times more likely to suffer from a depressive illness than a control group.[1]

What about horror writers? Are we more or less affected? After all, we write the stories that make your knees quiver and your marrow melt. Surely focussing on dark themes only serves to make our anxiety worse? Posts on my social media feed scream, 'Yes!', but my science training shouts back even louder: 'Anecdotal!'

Keen to explore this idea further, I messaged my American colleague Brian Matthews, a psychologist and the author of the *Forever Man* series of books. I suggested putting together a panel called 'Writing from a Dark Place' for an upcoming horror convention. Did Brian think a discussion of this nature was timely? Could the topic be addressed with sensitivity in a panel setting? Wasn't it interesting, I asked him, that so many of our horror icons, like Stephen King, Clive Barker, Mary Shelley, Edgar Allen Poe and even the poet Sylvia Plath, had all suffered with mental illness at one time or another? Brian responded with enthusiasm. I had my first panellist.

But how would we invite people with personal stories of anxiety and depression to join the panel? Dropping someone a line and asking, 'Hey, I heard you were depressed. Want to share?' wasn't going to cut it. What if the subject was too triggering?

---

[1] Kay Redfield Jamison, 'Manic-Depressive Illness and Creativity', *Scientific American* 272, no. 2 (Feb 1995): 62–67.

'We need to allow for flexibility,' I wrote in a later email to Brian. 'And have a few substitutes in the wings. Because you never know when the black dog will decide to sit on someone's face.'

We sifted through our contacts, invited some panellists, and sent off our proposal.

It was accepted.

A few months later I was at the Biltmore Hotel in Lovecraft's Providence, Rhode Island. Along with Brian and myself, our panellists were James Arthur Anderson, Eric Guignard, Brian Kirk and Leslie Klinger.[2] The event was scheduled for the end of the day, and I was nervous. Already that day, I had moderated two panels and appeared on another, but this one was personal. I went back to my room and tried to calm myself by browsing for puppies on the internet. It was no use; I was still nervous. I gave up and headed downstairs to hover in the corridor outside the conference suite. Would anyone turn up?

But my worrying was for nothing: participants of the previous session departed and the room filled in minutes.

My panellists came prepared to do all the heavy lifting. My colleague Brian Matthews started the session by talking about psychology. Neuro-imaging techniques, he explained, reveal that depressed or anxious people are unable to deactivate activity in the right precuneus of the brain, and that then acts on the amygdala, which results in more negative imaging activity.[3] Simply put, anxiety means that the brain is seldom at rest: we can't switch off our negative thinking.

Brian went further, explaining that the same rumination

---

2   Anderson, James Arthur, Eric Guignard, Brian Kirk, Leslie Klinger, Brian Matthews and Lee Murray, 'Writing from a Dark Place: Writing from Depression, Trauma and Grief', at StokerCon, Providence, Rhode Island, 2 March 2018 (comments confirmed by email).

3   Susan Nolen-Hoeksema, Blair E. Wisco and Sonja Lyubomirsky, 'Rethinking Rumination', *Association for Psychological Science* 3, no. 5 (2008): 400–24.

activity can be observed for the creative acts of editing and revising. I wanted to pump my fist in the air. Brian's comment had confirmed my suspicions: the wolf under the bed paces on and on, and even our physiology demands that we press our ears to the pillow to listen.

I thought of the famous quote by doctor and poet William Carlos Williams: 'All writing is a disease. You can't stop it.'

But lack of rest takes its toll, and some creative people turn to substance abuse to dampen the suffering, terrified that stifling their anxiety might stem the flow of ideas.

Stephen King is one example. James Arthur Anderson, who wrote *The Linguistics of Stephen King*, said that one reason King couldn't stop abusing cocaine and alcohol was because 'he was afraid that if he stopped the destructive behaviour, he wouldn't be able to write.' Brian Kirk, author of *We Are Monsters*, agreed. 'When artists venture deep into darkness,' he said, 'they typically suffer, whereas the art flourishes.'

'And yet,' Anderson said, 'after a serious intervention from his family, King was able to get clean, and his writing didn't suffer.' Anderson reminded us of a 2006 interview in which King drew an analogy between taking drugs and writing. 'I'm like a drug addict,' King had said. 'I'm always saying that I'm going to stop [writing], and then I can't. When I'm not working, my mind doesn't take kindly to being unhooked from its dope. I get migraines and very vivid nightmares . . . like my mind and body are trying to scare me back to work.'[4]

Brian pointed out that the act of writing *can* reduce activity in the part of the brain responsible for emotions. It's the rumination that's destructive. 'We just have to give ourselves permission to write badly,' he said.

Leslie Klinger, author of *The New Annotated H.P. Lovecraft* and *The New Annotated Frankenstein*, made a statement that

---

4 Nigel Farndale, 'I Want to Share My Nightmares', *Telegraph*, 12 November 2006.

gave us all pause. He said that, in his experience, writing nonfiction involves less rumination because the aim is to present factual information. I had to agree: it's harder to beat yourself up over a fact. Fiction, by contrast, seems more personal. When I'm writing fiction, where so much is conjured from my own experience, it's as if there is nowhere to hide.

Perhaps there's an upside to all my anxiety: if I'm continuously sifting and sorting ideas, testing and retesting theories, I might chance upon a new concept, perhaps even a new world. There's comfort in thinking that there might be a pay-off for reliving so many conversations in my head—even if it's only to make my characters' dialogue more interesting. And then there are those *eureka* moments, when you work out how to fill the gaping plot hole in your narrative, for example.

'One question that nagged me all the way through the writing process was: *How the hell am I going to kill the Karanadon?*' said Australian author Matthew Reilly in an interview about his alien thriller *Contest*. The answer came to him 'completely out of the blue. It just hit me. I started dancing around the house, pumping my fists in the air.'[5]

Nancy C. Andreasen, Chair of Psychiatry at the University of Iowa, wrote her seminal paper on the topic of creativity, and observed that while many creative people 'suffer from mood and anxiety disorders, they associate their gifts with strong feelings of joy and excitement.'[6] On our panel, Kirk made a similar observation. 'There is a kind of polarity coded into the natural order of the world,' he said. 'It takes darkness to perceive light. Therefore, to create something beautiful, like a work of art, it must be counterbalanced. Unfortunately, that counterweight appears to be suffering commonly expressed through anxiety, depression, obsessive disorders.'

---

5   'In Interview with Matthew Reilly', *Contest* (Australia: Pan MacMillan, 2007).
6   Nancy C. Andreasen, 'Secrets of the Creative Brain', *Atlantic*, July/August 2014.

But why, then, do we write horror? Surely dark subjects only serve to make us more morose. Why not write light-hearted stories?

'Because facing the darkness often leads to great art,' said Kirk. 'And the deeper we venture, the better it gets.'

I knew what he meant. I started out writing chick-lit, and while readers of my work found the stories fun, I quickly lost interest. The characters weren't challenging enough for me, their conflicts too banal. It's hard to conjure up emotional depth when you're writing characters whose biggest crises involve cupcake deprivation and wardrobe malfunctions.

On our panel, Eric Guignard, horror short fiction specialist, suggested that dark fiction is a means of 'probing, through action, or interaction with others, the effects of varying conditions and scenarios with which to overcome the bleakness.' True enough, I thought. If we've prepared our survival route in our heads, then it follows that when the zombie apocalypse comes, we're going to be better equipped to survive. Plus, if we write for long enough, there is always the hope that we might be rewarded with more of those rare, joyful, eureka moments.

When our panel discussion was over, we opened the session to comments from the floor. The discussion was frank. People talked about self-care and about what it was like to write while on medication. Nicole Cushing, author of *The Sadist's Bible*, raised her hand and told us that a few years ago she had been diagnosed with Obsessive Compulsive Disorder and prescribed sertraline (the generic for Zoloft). 'When I first started taking the pills, I noticed a difference in how my brain was working,' she said. 'At first it felt like my brain had been put on a leash. Which was okay. It needed one, given the near-paranoia I was suffering. Over time, though, I came to realise that the leash metaphor was incorrect. It was more like my brain was a car that had fallen into disrepair, and for decades I had procrastinated in getting it fixed.

And when things finally got so bad that I had to get help, and I let people help me, the repairs were done and I found that my brain handled more smoothly than I ever thought possible. It's like I didn't have the ability to know what true mental health felt like, because I had never experienced it. I just assumed everyone's brains worked like mine did, in the same way that some people get so used to driving with poorly inflated tyres or failing brakes or one headlight that they don't notice it. They only notice how much better things are when those issues get fixed.'

Back home in New Zealand, I messaged Cushing to thank her for her contribution, and I asked her if writing horror helps her push back the darkness.

She replied, 'For me, there is a sense of mastery that comes from using fiction to look my deepest, darkest demons in the eye. To look at traumatic events, and not flinch from them, and then capture them in the cage of a novel feels like a victory.'

Capture them in the cage of a novel.

Her words made me think of my yellow-eyed wolf, pacing and panting beneath my bed. I wrote about him once. In the story, my tiny protagonist stabs the wolf with a pocket knife but is unable to kill him.[7]

I understand now that my wolf can't be killed. Instead, I will let him stalk me in the darkness, and then, one day, I will capture him in the cage of a novel.

---

7   Lee Murray, 'Peter and the Wolf', in *Baby Teeth: Bite-sized Tales of Terror*, ed. Dan Rabarts and Lee Murray (Wellington: Paper Road Press), 196.

Moving Earth

Selina Tusitala Marsh

A friend said I didn't belong in this book. 'You're the least depressed person I know!' I was struck by her incredulity and the finality with which she spoke about my impossible citizenship in the land of the lost, the pained, the anxious, the depressed, the stuck. What I heard was: *Look at you! You're the goddamn Poet Laureate. You met President Obama two weeks ago, the Queen two years ago. You'll probably meet Oprah next year. And you're running a trail marathon next week!*

I could've laughed it off, taken it on the chin. After all, I'm not on medication; I haven't ever been told that I am depressed; I don't have to live with a debilitating, life-threatening illness; I can eat like a horse and run like one if I have to. What do I have to be anxious about? Like, not just day-to-day anxious, as in, 'Shite, Arianna Huffington! I still can't get more than six hours sleep a night! Yikes, I have back-to-back meetings and parent-teacher interviews for the next three days! Flip, the book deadline is at the same time as my exam marking, two overseas festivals, an article and four scheduled community workshops! Faaar out.' I mean, anxious enough to contribute to this book.

Still. As well as my friend knows me, she also doesn't. While she's seen my many sides, she isn't intimate with the prism shadows I've lived with all my life. Those tiny refracted moments that skew perspective. I remember being 12, and while staring at my reflection in the stainless-steel playground slide my dad had left behind after he'd left us all, wondering whether I was depressed. Then, by logical deduction, I dismissed it. I didn't look like the TV show characters who were depressed. I didn't have a sad-looking face or a sad voice or sad clothes. I loved laughing and making others laugh. I was loud on the outside, but always aware of an unsounded space, an isolation, a deep feeling of difference, of pressing my nose against the glass and looking in.

Like how people treated me and my sister. Sam is four years younger than me, and as a kid she had straight brown hair and gorgeous big brown eyes petalled by the darkest lashes. She was very, very cute. I was too tall and thin, with wild wiry hair. Mum would parade us out to show her friends, and we would stand side by side. 'Oh, you're so beautiful,' Mum's friends would coo to my sister. 'You should be a model!' Then, as if seeing me for the first time: 'And . . . why, you're so . . . tall!'

I remember going next door to play on the neighbours' swing-set with Helen, a girl who was Sam's age and who wore her hair like my sister too, in enviable ribboned pigtails. (I couldn't wear pigtails—they came out like earmuff pompoms.) We were having fun until Helen's mother said I was too big to play with the younger girls and perhaps I should go home. I crawled through the bordering hedge, humiliated. That feeling of being on the outside has followed me around.

I think I'm a high-functioning anxious person. Like my dad, a high-functioning alcoholic, people would never know it or suspect it: I hide it well. I'm happy *and* anxious. You can be both, and I have excellent coping mechanisms. Running, for example. I have so much on my plate right now that my monthly planner looks like a plate of neon-coloured spaghetti that's been knocked over. But I've just signed up for the Waitomo Trail Run—I'll be running an underground-overground 22-kilometre trail on Saturday—and the 19-kilometre Tongariro Crossing on the Sunday. I have to run. I can't lie in bed at 4:45a.m. angsting over whether I have 45 minutes in the 14-hour work day ahead to run; I just get up and run. The most anxiety-relieving kind of run is in the bush in my Vibram toe shoes—a.k.a. Zoe Saldana's feet in *Avatar*; freaky but strangely sexy, are they not?—listening to Adam Lambert's remix of 'If I Can't Have You', with my hair out. This morning I burst out of the bush on to the road, hair and music in full swing, nearly knocking a guy in a hi-vis vest holding a Stop/Go sign off his feet. 'Whoa!' he shouted. 'You just let it all hang out, girl!'

I shouted over my shoulder, 'That's wild hair bush-runnin' man!'

I've come to know that for me, stillness, unless it's mindful, is a slippery slope into the Void. At least, into one part of it—the airless part, where everything and everyone, even colours and textures, are too much for me to handle. The multiple, continuous, simultaneous demands are too high, and in response, I freeze. My breathing is bare and shallow. The tips of my fingers go numb. I climb into the cave of my bed and, unsounded, I stay there.

Like I did after Mum died. No one knew I was in my cave. I would get out of bed to get the family out the door, go back to bed, then get up before the family returned. I'd lay out my laptop, scatter the books, make coffee then empty it into the sink. It looked as if I'd been working on my book, marking essays, prepping classes all day.

One morning, deep inside my cave, I got a text from Jules: 'Yo—u cmg to kbxing?' She'd told me about this gym on the island, this kick-boxing champ-turned-trainer, how she and the girls just love it. She kept hassling me to come, sending weekly text reminders. Finally, after staring at the lit screen one day, I just went. I got out of bed, put on a T-shirt and tights, and got in the car and drove.

That's where my second collection of poetry, *Dark Sparring*, came from. To get through the death of my mum to breast cancer, I took up kick-boxing. Moving unblocked me. I learned to punch for the first time. To kick and block, grapple and wrestle. I'd never been with people, or myself, like this before.

I was grateful. I had somewhere to do battle with this lonely, unsounded thing within me. In the ring the rules are different; it's a heady mixture of self and others, a dance and play of bodies and minds. That was in 2009.

I've found other ways of moving through my anxiety. Even here, halfway through this essay, I hear my friend's voice. *You're too happy! You're way too giving and caring and community oriented! You're way too successful; you're the best at everything and now here you are, trying to be the best at anxiety.* Okay, so maybe that's not completely *her* voice, but . . . Oh, and there's the unsounded thing again, and here I am crawling back through the neighbour's hedge and into my cave.

Last year, I got my first stalker. There were over a thousand emails, midnight hang-up calls, threatening communications, even defacement of my property. I saw a workplace counsellor for the first time. I wasn't sleeping properly and began checking comms at all hours to see whether there was yet another deranged message left. My dreams were filling up with crazy funhouse mirror reflections of warped faces, elongated intonations of complaint and accusation.

I was randomly paired with an Indian clinical psychologist, and we clicked. As brown women succeeding in a Pākehā-led society, we began exhuming buried stories in socio-political-cultural-historical terrain. These were the stories that questioned our right to 'be'. I mind-mapped a lot. I drew a lot. The psychologist even photocopied my session notes with my permission because they were so creative and engaged. (*There you go again, you just have to be the best!*) She gave me permission to be extremely successful as well as extremely human and extremely self-compassionate.

As part of a university research project to do with voice and writing, I've been working with Sylvia Rands, an actor, voice coach and teacher of a concept called 'the sacred feminine'. Ostensibly, these voice lessons are to help me figure out any connections between audible and written voices. But I hadn't expected that, when learning how to sound out earth, water, fire and air, I would be sounding the source of my anxiety.

As a poet and performer, I reign in the air and fire modes. I occupy, manifest and project. Onstage I'm in my power—legs astride, arms akimbo, hair flying (what Amy Cuddy, author of *Presence*, calls the 'superhero pose'). What I'm not so good at is letting people know when I'm disappointed or upset, or, God forbid, angry. Formative childhood experiences taught me that these emotions aren't acceptable and make you unworthy of being let through the hedge again.

Earth is where the anger sits. It is raw and real. It says 'F*ck the world; this is me, this is what I feel and know to be true. F*ck people-pleasing, toe-licking, self-doubting, kowtowing. F*ck you. And f*ck me for having given a f*ck.' (It's no coincidence that I have three books by Sarah Knight—who wrote *Get Your Sh*t Together* and *The Life-Changing Magic of Not Giving a F*ck*—beside my bed.) Earth tone is black stone deep, the volcano's underbelly where you find the rock facts.

When Sylvia asked how my week had gone (and I think she meant how had the practice exercises gone, and those exercises are hard because they involve lubricating rusty vocal cords through sound, volume and tone, and neighbours don't appreciate hearing *AAAAMMMMMMMHEEEEEEEEERRRRRREEEEEEEE* at full volume at 6:30a.m.) I told her about my most humiliating Wednesday.

A well-known Pacific Island fashion house had contacted me and wanted to know if they could dress me for the Obama event. I had previously worn their beautiful dresses to events, most notably a puletasi (Samoan-styled dress) to perform for the Queen. I bought these dresses at full price, and mentioned them in a poem in support of Pacific people. Photographs of me, the dress and the Queen were featured on the front page of newspapers in New Zealand, throughout the Pacific and

Europe. The fashion house shared these images on their social media. Feeling like Cinderella, I went and tried out a number of dresses and finally chose one. I was then asked for my credit card. I was shocked. And speechless. And shamed that I had thought this was a gift in the Pacific spirit of reciprocity. The price of the dress I'd chosen was not in my budget, but to save face I bought another one on sale. They said they'd happily loan me the other dress. I agreed, and exited the shop red-faced. I rang my friend. She was outraged—but I was not. I was running out with an Eftpos receipt dragging between my legs. I was anxious—in the first place because my assumption was so embarrassing and that I felt I had to save face by buying my dignity back; and in the second place because my earth voice had crumbled so abysmally and, wet with my tears, become voiceless sludge.

With Sylvia, I practised my earth tone, first without words. Guttural, rusty, deep. 'HAAAAAA ... HAAAAA ... HAAAAA.'

'What are you thinking and feeling now, Selina?'

'Um, that I hope I'm doing it right, Sylvia?'

'Fuck Sylvia, Selina! This is about you. Honour you.'

'HAAAAAA ... HAAAAA ... HAAAAA.'

The sounds weren't pretty, not even powerful, but they began to be real. Then we practised with words, each word rising deep from within till it exploded, not in high sparks, but in a flaming flow of thick, hot lava, each word accompanied by heel to earth movement and a calling forth swing of the arms: 'I ... AM ... WORTHY' and 'I ... HAVE ... EARNED ... RESPECT'.

Then the release came. I let go of worrying about what others might think and whether I was doing my life right. I contacted the fashion house and explained why I felt humiliated, how when the Māori designer Jeanine Clarkin from Waiheke had dressed me she'd given me the dress in return for being her walking billboard on the international stage. It seemed like the pono thing to do. They apologised for the misunderstanding. They said if they were in a better financial position they would've given me the dress. I thanked them for their apology.

My friend is still appalled, but I've said my piece. I'm learning to cope with my anxiety around my feeling of voicelessness, which many might find surprising (*What? You're the goddamn Poet Laureate!*). I'm still practising Sylvia's exercises. I move my voice through earth to water to fire to air, like moving my body through trail, through bush, through rock, through cave, like moving my pen into story and my voice into sound.

Sit in the Fire

Jess McAllen

Last year, I shared my room with mice. The flat, a 100-year-old Wellington house with salmon walls and a landlord who would turn up unannounced, was $175 a week including expenses. My flatmates were creative—an actor, a makeup artist, a student artist with a penis candle, a comedian—and for a year we made a big talk of resuscitating the damp lounge. The kitchen ceiling peeled from the leaking shower in the room above. A mushroom grew in the bathroom. Later, a frazzled property manager would tell us we hadn't even been on the lease. It was my second year freelancing—which mostly meant working from bed, under the blankets and alone for long periods of time, compulsively messaging friends at their full-time jobs. Who would've guessed freelancing isn't ideal for a person with mental health issues? Turns out, everyone. My friends, family, former workmates and old psychiatrist warned against it, but I persisted. The year I shared my room with mice was the year of my third breakdown.

    I was 14 when I had my first breakdown. If you go by depictions in popular media, you could say I'd lost my mind. I would stay up until three o'clock, terrified to go to bed, reading until my eyelids moved like a drunk jackhammer and I could start to make out a kaleidoscope of faces in the curtains, big and small and weird, until passing out. Falling asleep like this beat the alternative: getting out of bed over and over to check there wasn't a murderer in my wardrobe and pushing down on the window locks until callouses appeared on my fingertips. There started my journey with the public mental health system.

Apparently too batshit for a private counsellor, who'd initially tried to pin it down to depression, I was referred urgently to Infant Child and Adolescent Mental Health Services (ICAMHS). ICAMHS is a publicly funded service that provides assessment and treatment for children and teenagers with 'moderate to severe mental health problems', according to the Waikato DHB website. It took six months for me to get an appointment with a psychiatrist, but once I was there she taught me about different forms of anxiety. It wasn't just the stock-standard hyperventilating into a paper bag. It was those moments when my stomach squeezed itself and I zoned out—these, I was told, were panic attacks. There was relief in the diagnosis, knowing that the bizarre and endless thought-loops wouldn't necessarily land me in hospital. Hearing the symptoms rattled off by the psychiatrist and understanding why my previous diagnosis of depression didn't quite explain everything helped. Around this time, things got so bad that I lived with my aunty for a bit in Foxton Beach, and upon returning home I was greeted with the antidepressant fluoxetine. At seventeen, the symptoms stopped and I vowed never to let myself get to that point again. For a while, anxiety largely stayed away. It felt like I had won.

Depression dominated my early 20s, and, soon after graduating university, I became suicidal. I went into the public system again. It was a different battle this time—I just wanted to die. Again, there was a months-long wait to see a psychiatrist through the public system, and due to the long wait I was halfway through my treatment when I started my first journalism job in May 2014. That was when I learnt that, for many people who have mental health issues, you don't just have one bout of depression or anxiety and then get over it. Recovery is more about how you manage the recurring types of mental health issues and learn to live your life around them.

In 2017, during my third breakdown, the anxiety came back in a different form from what I'd experienced as a teenager, such that it took months for me to recognise it had reared its head again. The depression and suicidal ideation was there as well, but thankfully I never felt as desperately suicidal as I had in late 2013 and early 2014.

Suicide and mental health were constantly in the news, largely thanks to the 2017 election, when many of the flaws in the public mental health system were drawn to attention and used to score political points. Nearly every day there was another news story proclaiming to know the system—the loudest people talking, of course, weren't using the public mental health system themselves; they were usually advocates of their family members or friends. A union campaign toured 606 pairs of shoes across the country, each pair representing a New Zealander who had died by suicide. On 10 September the union and bereaved families they had teamed up with arrived at Parliament and laid out the hundreds of pairs of shoes to commemorate World Suicide Prevention Day. There were dozens of news stories as a result. It all became very intense and, to me, it wasn't representative of the nuances of the mental health system. It made me reflect on my experience, the times I'd been let down and at real risk, and the times when the public system probably saved me.

I'd had one psychiatrist who liked Freud and theorised that my love of reading was in the name of impressing my parents, both of whom are English teachers. There was the one who, when I googled him, was named for dismissing a patient who then went on to murder someone (his relative would later email my journalism address, pitching stories about the need to get rid of the insanity plea). There was the caseworker who gave me her personal cellphone number when I needed it most. There was the mindfulness course I took at age 21, two hours a week with others who'd recently attempted suicide, to tide us over until a psychologist was available (by the time I was near the top of the eight-month waiting list, I'd moved to a different catchment zone and had to start on a new waiting list).

Last year I went through Te Haika, Wellington's free mental health service. Earlier, I had attended the entry appointment, during which you outline your problems to a social worker and the team then decide whether or not to accept you. That I'd had two previous stints with specialist mental health swung things in my favour, but I know many people who have needed help and been turned away. But I was lucky: a month or so later, I was assigned a psychiatrist. We played around with my medications and my case worker told me that the physical act of smiling can sometimes help beat a bad mood. Eight months later I started my first therapy appointment in 10 years. This was when the help really started.

This psychologist asked what could be causing stress in my life: was it work, was it my home life? Could I even tell the difference anymore? I thought about my house, its thigh-high grass in the backyard and the cardboard cut-out of Max from *Where the Wild Things Are* which stood at the top of the stairs. My bedroom, the floor of which sloped slightly down towards the fireplace so I couldn't help but roll when getting into bed. The big window that looked out to tall pine trees and a faded New World sign. The fireplace, sellotaped over with tinfoil. The way the mice had a little hole they could get through. The dress, found in a cupboard, that was rolled up to stuff the hole.

I'd tried to channel my anxious energy into the family of mice who lived in the fireplace in my room. At times they would jump through the tinfoil cover we'd fashioned and run around squeaking. I'd tack peanut butter onto a large plastic container to lure them out, but in the last second they'd always manage to nip a bite and dart back. One winter night, when I was no longer able to sleep in my bed without imagining the mice running over me, I tried to sleep on a damp couch in the lounge instead and I realised the mice had to die. I left them a last tasty treat, a slice of four-dollar camembert and set a trap. My flatmate dealt with the remains.

Like most people's anxiety, mine stems from a need to take some control in an unpredictable world. In retrospect, my panic around the mice was less a hatred for the creatures than my fear of what they represented: I couldn't stop my mental health problems from coming out of the dark fireplace. And I couldn't afford to move to a new place.

Part of my therapy is exposure. My psychologist tells me that, to stop checking on things and seeking reassurance, you have to sit with the anxiety. There's a popular online meme you may have seen of a dog drinking a cup of coffee while flames burn around him, his speech bubble saying, 'This is fine.' People have repurposed the meme all over the internet, applying it to Trump or to climate change, but for me it means exposure therapy.

We make a list and rank all the things I'm worried about: mice, intruders. Constantly having to check the locks on my bedroom door and window is exhausting, and the anxieties feed into each other and spiral. Most have roots in trauma. I can live my life and go years without some of these anxieties, so when they come back it's frustrating when they affect my ability to sleep and write. They're a telltale sign that something isn't right in my life, that I need a method to deal with this thing and exert some control.

The goal, my psychologist says, is to be okay with leaving my second-storey bedroom window open at night. Immediately I laugh, but secretly I wish to do this. For my anxiety, medication isn't always enough: after my first two years on it, the effect seemed to peter out. To be okay with the fact that the world is inherently risky is the real goal.

My psychologist and I sit in the addictions building near the hospital, because the mental health building was damaged in the Kaikōura earthquake. He tries to drum in to me that you can take all the precautions in the world and you still aren't safe. The rooms are often overheated but they have the best mental-health art (flowers, oceans) that I've seen. It occurs to me that picking art for mental-health buildings probably isn't a very fun task—they don't want to overstimulate us. In the reception, the workers are protected behind windows. It makes me feel like a threat, as I grab the free fruit they provide on Wednesdays.

My psychologist holds his clipboard and there's a folder on the table. It is filled with little tests I've taken, forms like *Rate the past week* and *What are your core values?* I'm allowed to keep the sheets that are interesting; the ones on radical acceptance and unhelpful thinking patterns live next to my hair straightener. My therapist knows I write about mental health for a living, and, unlike other professionals, he doesn't get an annoyed look when I know the terminology. We talk about articles we've read.

There's a logical answer for every concern, he tells me, but anxiety favours those with overactive imaginations. If there's someone hiding under the bed, my psychiatrist asks, why would they stay there for so long—wouldn't they immediately make themselves known? He sits with his legs crossed, trying to out-logic me. But, I tell him, I read about a man who lived in an attic all year and then attacked the family below.

It's my turn to question him: what if someone accidentally leaves the oven on?

Fire alarm, he shoots back.

What if a mouse crawls over me while I sleep?

That's gross, he agrees. But that's also life.

These back and forths often end in laughter. I know how ridiculous I sound—in fact, sometimes this makes it all the more painful, the constant refrain of someone trying to reason with anxiety.

He tells me about people with different types of extreme anxiety. A common worry of people with obsessive compulsive disorder is feeling guilty—like, if you don't touch a door three times, you will cause an earthquake. It's quite hard to reason with that in an earthquake-prone city like Wellington. There are the mothers who can't touch their own children, such are their contamination fears, he says. There's the fear of hitting someone when driving and having to double back multiple times. Mental illness has taken away so much from so many, and it serves to remember that I could have it a lot worse.

Eight months since I first started seeing the psychologist, I'm in a better flat and in a better financial position. I still have anxiety (and other mental health issues), but the stability of being able to pay rent and having a sunny, mouse-free room makes sitting with the anxiety more achievable. I feel privileged in this regard: my experience trying to get a benefit last year was exhausting, and I gave up. Mental health is affected so profoundly by how much money you have and where you live. People who can't get by day-to-day become even more vulnerable.

These days, when I'm in the fire I try to see how long I can sit in it. Putting it out may be a temporary relief, but if I keep doing that, it will just come back. Instead, on good days, I sit in it and feel the flames lick at me, there but not always burning.

The Midst

Allan Drew

The first time I had a panic attack, I was running. This is true and untrue.

I was on the corner of Mt Eden Road and Balmoral Road on a winter afternoon. I was training for a marathon. Marathon training is a good thing, and a bad thing (marathons are miserable and humiliating, but in a good way). On that corner I stopped running, hunched over, shook, and began to cry—for the simple reason that my wife was being murdered.

I've said it was my first panic attack. It wasn't. It was just the first time I labelled the experience as a panic attack—or rather the first time someone else gave my experience that label. It was my wife, still living, who informed me of this when she came to pick me up.

I stumbled, sobbing and convulsing, and still sweating from running, into a service station on Balmoral Road and asked to use their phone. The guy behind the counter said I couldn't—it wasn't policy—but then he relented. I guess it was because of how I looked. I made the call, hung up, then bawled without control outside on the footpath while my wife drove out to get me. You've had a panic attack, she said, in all her unmurdered glory.

But no, on reflection, not my first. I've been having them all my life. Off and on, here and there.

In my early days of university I learned about the term *in medias res*, or 'in the midst of things'. Some stories begin in the middle of the narrative, before regressing to fill in the blanks. This is how I began this essay, and also how I began my experience with mental illness. I came to define the problem suddenly, at a distinct moment, and yet I've had the problem for as long as I could remember. Perhaps there is nothing quite as *in medias res* as a mental health diagnosis. Does it go like this for everyone?

Mental health professional: 'You're mentally ill.'

Person [thinking, remembering, knowing—having always known]: 'Oh. Really? Okay.'

The trigger for a panic attack is both critical and irrelevant. In the moment, the trigger is everything, and all you can think of is eliminating it. The reality is that in the absence of *that* trigger it would have been something else. I've always felt my anxiety, at its worst, to be free-floating and adhesive: it latches on to anything. The trigger when I was out on that run was having left my wife at home when someone was coming over to deliver a washing machine. That person, in my absence, would murder her. She was pregnant with our daughter at the time. That was eight years ago.

You might think that my panic was altruistic—that I was worried about the safety of my wife and child. But that wasn't it—not to my mind. It was *my own* safety that was at risk. Without a wife and daughter, there would be nothing for me. *I* would be alone. *I* would be unsafe. When I realised my selfishness, it made it worse. Such is the spiral of anxiety; such is the trap.

That panic attack wasn't, as it turns out, when I truly took on my diagnosis. It was a landmark moment only in retrospect.

My wife and I use a numerical scale to test my mood. If I say I'm 10, it means I'm well. Not necessarily blissful (although I might be), but well. I might have had a crappy day, be overwhelmed by work, have a backache or diarrhoea, and have ranted about the cricket, but I'm still 10, still 100% well. At my worst I was a zero. I remember saying it: 'I'm zero,' and I remember thinking I would have substituted that feeling with anything else. Extreme physical pain would have been a relief.

If cutting off my arm would have cured me, I wouldn't have hesitated. Strange thoughts give rise to strange thoughts, and so the cycle goes on. When I was low, my job was to wait.

I'm using the past tense to talk about this thing, because I'm currently at a 10, and have been thereabouts for some years. Thanks to the lessons of time and experience, I feel more capable. But back then, when low, my job was simply to wait. Lorazepam helped. Sleep helped. Time passes, and the passage of time is such a strong source of hope. I feel like it's its own entity, and that it deserves its own word: time-promise.

When our daughter was two weeks old I began crying at the kitchen bench while cutting an apple. Something was terribly wrong, but I didn't know what. I'd had not much sleep, of course, and my life had changed beyond recognition in only a few days. Looking back now, I feel like I should have seen it coming.

We've planted a flowering cherry tree in the backyard, and in September I can stand in the garden and breathe it in, and it's hard to feel anything other than happy in that moment. Lemon blossom is the best. I shove my face in lemon flowers when I can, and will pick them if no one is watching (people will always tell you, even though you know, that the flowers become fruit). I scrunch the picked flowers in my fingers, and the fragrant oil absorbs into my skin. The smell stays for hours. I do the same with eucalyptus leaves, grabbing handfuls when I go on a run, snapping the leaves and squeezing out the sticky fluid. This is what I think happens: the smell goes directly to my limbic system, to my evolutionarily ancient brainstem. I had a teacher who called the brainstem the 'lizard brain'. In firing up my lizard brain, the scent bypasses, or short-circuits, my prefrontal cortex, where my anxiety fizzes.

It took Satan nine days and nine nights to fall from the kingdom of heaven into the dungeon of hell. So says John Milton in *Paradise Lost*. When Satan awoke after his fall, he stood, brushed himself off, and said to his companions, 'Here at least we shall be free.' That line has become a refrain for me. It's not that I identify with Satan, or think my existence anything approximating hell. It just seems a remarkably optimistic utterance in that situation. Plus, I love that poem. Milton's Satan is one of literature's greatest, and most resilient, optimists.

I say it all the time to myself—*here at least we shall be free*—including in situations where it's not appropriate: in queues at the post office, when stuck in traffic, at funerals, weddings, while swimming, in my dreams. I wrote a story about my granddad, who rowed his dinghy to visit a US destroyer anchored in Mercury Bay during World War 2. He stroked the oars to the iambic rhythm of that phrase. *Here at least we shall be free; here at least we shall be free.*

Paradise Lost is the literary version of lemon blossom. I can't scrunch it in my fingers, but it zips to my lizard brain nonetheless.

When our daughter was two weeks old, and I starting crying in the kitchen, I didn't know about lemon blossom, and I didn't know about Milton's poem. The time-promise brought these to me. My job was to wait, and to let time pass. It took a few months. My psychiatrist said to try fluoxetine, and to give it time to work. I did, and it did. From what I can tell, I'm one of the lucky ones for whom selective serotonin reuptake inhibitors make a real difference. But I think these drugs are often poorly understood by people who don't take them. They don't make me feel euphoric, and they don't stop me from caring about anything. They help me to feel like I can deal with difficult things better.

I can't remember my psychiatrist's name. It's in my phone, probably. He was a strange man. He prescribed me so many pills along with fluoxetine. Lorazepam, zopiclone, quetiapine. I have a container filled with the remains of these pills. I tried them all, with variable success. Someone told me that quetiapine is known on the street as Suzie Q and is used recreationally to smooth out a rough high. All it ever did for me was put me to sleep during a rough low. Zopiclone gave me hangovers, the worst part of which was a persistent and foul metallic taste. Lorazepam is like having three or four beers. Fluoxetine, on the other hand, had no noticeable effect for a while, but in the end, it woke me up.

My trigger was easy to define: I was worried about our newborn daughter's sleep patterns. I'd read that new babies are supposed to sleep about 16 hours a day, but she was only sleeping 10.5 hours. I knew because I kept a spreadsheet tracking her overnight sleep and her daytime naps. Various people have said this was a classic example of the hypervigilance of anxiety, although learning this word didn't really help. (She still sleeps about that much. That's what she needs.)

I tried a few therapists, and they were always good people. They said my anxiety about my daughter's sleep was an extension of a natural feeling. I knew that, of course, and it's that tether to reality that makes anxiety so difficult to deal with. Pathological anxiety is the unhelpful, alarmist cousin of rational concern. Therapy helped me, but not when things were bad. In the middle of a crisis, cognitive therapy is like a turning a garden hose on a forest fire. But those techniques can really help when things are just beginning to smoulder.

Anxiety is never simple. It was true that I was concerned for my daughter's development, but part of the reason I felt so bad was that I was worried about how my daughter's lack of sleep would affect *me*—how I would be able to make it through in an ongoing state of exhaustion. Just like during that panic attack on Balmoral Road eight years ago, I had that same sense of self-loathing. It both begins and perpetuates the downward spiral.

But you can spiral up, too: it's part of the time-promise. I recently came across an argument in a thesis I was proofreading.

The student spent thousands of words explaining that the word 'recovery' is the wrong word to use for mental illness. Instead, she preferred 'recovering', because recovering is a process of living that just carries on. The concept appeals to me because it's so very *in medias res*, so very *in the midst of things*. Part of me says it's kind of bullshit, too, because it's just swapping a noun for a verb and claiming an insight; it also suggests that you'll never truly get better, like you'll never be *recovered*. On the other hand, it's not bullshit at all: how do you recover from your own brain? I'm five feet, nine inches tall (five-nine-and-a-half in the morning, before gravity gets to me): I can't shake that biological fact. In some ways I'll always be 'recovering' from my mediocre height, but in other ways the process of recovering is learning to accept that that's how things are—and that's part of spiralling up.

My wife and I have absorbed our numbering system into daily life. When we talk about our days, she'll often ask, 'Number?' I answer almost always with '10.' Not everyone has such supportive people they can call on, and I know that for some, even those who have strong support, it's not always enough. I know I'm lucky. My daughter, whose entry into the world I was unable to deal with rationally for a while, is now the surest source of joy. She's better than any scrunched-up lemon flower, any eucalypt, any verse from Milton. Time passes; she changes; but she also remains the same: she's the best manifestation of the time-promise, of a life *in medias res*. It's the easiest thing in the world to say, when next to her, 'Here at least we shall be free.'

My Geography

Yvette Walker

In 2014, my wife and I went for a day trip to Bath, in Somerset. It was a rainy June day. We parked the car at the Bath Cricket Club, walked into the city, wound our way through the shopping precinct and then tramped uphill towards the famous Circus. On the way I bought an antique watch, a lovely example of British watchmaking from between the Wars. The watch was a little bumped and bruised but was still in good working order. We met my wife's cousin Tim and his partner, Sally, in a large cafe, which was fitted out like a grocer crossed with a greenhouse. We ordered cake and tea.

At some point during our conversation I thought that someone had turned the volume up. I looked around the room. It wasn't busy: there were maybe 20 people in the cafe, but the volume was approaching that Spinal Tap 11 on the dial. My palms started to sweat, and I couldn't breathe very well. The tastefully decorated walls seemed to be closing in on me. I looked at my wife, then at Tim and Sally. They seemed fine. Then I twigged: I was having a panic attack. I told my wife I was 'going outside for a bit'—code for 'I'm freaking out and I need to calm down'—and I stood up and walked out onto the cobbled street into the rain. As I walked away from the cafe I tried to remain calm and present, I tried to focus on each and every breath.

At the end of the street was a high-end art dealer. In the window was an 18th-century painting of an English gentleman, landed gentry I supposed, painted by a famous artist I had never heard of. I wondered what life would have to be like in order to be able to afford that painting, and, if I had that life, would I spend it on a painting like this one? Oddly enough, thinking about the lives of posh stockbrokers, League One footballers and Tory politicians helped to calm me down. The rain helped, too. Here I was, standing in the rain in Bath, staring in a shop window at a beautifully rendered portrait of an aristocrat. What could be wrong? Nothing was wrong.

Sometimes, anxiety doesn't seem to be made up of anything at all. Sometimes there is no inciting incident, no specific thing that flicks that switch. Anxiety can come to you in the most ordinary of moments.

I first met anxiety on my modest book tour for my debut novel. Cultivating the desire to be published, over years and years, sets you up for some odd emotional experiences once you are finally there, inside the circle. Anxiety is one of the experiences waiting for you. I found out quite quickly that performance anxiety is not uncommon among writers, both new and established. Casual chat in the green room or at the bar would inevitably turn to how to keep low-level anxiety from turning into blind terror. Some people exercised, some meditated, some drank, some blew off entire festivals and went somewhere else, did something else, until it was their session. Some took beta-blockers. I was surprised, and not surprised at the same time. A friend of mine, a cellist, told me she was doing her doctorate on the use of beta-blockers by classical musicians to overcome stage fright and performance anxiety. And my brother, an actor for over 20 years, confessed to me that he still got stage fright. Until it was me, sitting up on a stage, I hadn't given the emotional side of performance a second thought. I know from conversations with people afterwards that I don't appear nervous, or flustered—but it's just luck that I appear relaxed and at ease. The truth is a little more complicated.

Once, before a reading at the Wheeler Centre in Melbourne, I took refuge in a tiny bathroom. In the mirror, I could see a red bruise spreading across my neck and throat like a cartographer's mistake. I didn't know what it could be, and all I wanted was for it to stop, whatever it was. Didn't it know I had to go and do a public reading in half an hour? Oh, it knew. That's why it was there. I got through the reading by wrapping my grey scarf around the offending splotches and downing a martini afterwards. I was more bemused than concerned. Other readings and events were mostly okay; the red mark made an occasional appearance, but nothing else happened. But, towards the end of the tour, I started feeling ill. By the time I flew home to Western Australia, I was feeling incredibly nauseous.

Not long after that, early one Saturday morning, I ended up in Accident and Emergency with appendicitis. I'd had no localised pain in my abdomen, so I hadn't connected my persistent nausea to anything more sinister. The surgeons got to my appendix in the nick of time. Even though I developed post-surgery complications, at least I wasn't dead.

One Sunday afternoon, while I was still recovering, a good friend and her son came over for afternoon tea. We had tea and cake in the backyard, and it was lovely. And my wife was coming home to Perth from Sydney later that evening. But the minute after I had waved goodbye to my guests, the minute after I had gone inside and sat down, the world began to shake. Was it an earthquake? I had no other reference for what was happening. When I realised that it was me shaking and not the ground underneath me, I thought I must be having a heart attack. But my symptoms didn't stop, and I obviously wasn't having a cardiac arrest. I started googling.

I realised that what I was experiencing was a full-body panic attack and that it could last quite some time. My wife wouldn't be home for hours, and I was too embarrassed to call any of my friends. Somehow, I toughed it out. The attack lasted around 70 minutes. When it was over, I drank a litre of water and put myself to bed.

My doctor said that going under general anaesthetic could trigger post-operative panic attacks in some people, though no one knew why it happened. He prescribed propranolol, a mild, non-addictive beta-blocker that I could use when I needed to. I wondered whether it was the trauma of my almost burst appendix, playing out weeks later; or was it an older trauma that had broken its chains and journeyed to the surface of my conscious self? Or was the panic not coming from me at all? The world is a constant procession of calamity, violence and injustice; how could this fail to seep into a person's nervous system? Even if you shut yourself off and don't engage, it is still there—the constant hum of humanity failing.

I wondered whether a panic attack was simply the body's way of dealing with the accumulated stress of being in the world. Some kind of muddle-headed release mechanism. Were my panic attacks the faultline at which my personal biography met the world's biography? If the world was perfect tomorrow, would my panic end?

Probably not.

If you have ever had a panic attack, you may have, at some point, believed that you were to blame for it. But that's like saying it's your fault when you sneeze. It's true that, maybe, you shouldn't have walked home in the rain that day, or maybe you could have avoided that burst of spring pollen you walked past one sunny afternoon—but you know, in that moment, that the sneeze was beyond your control. No one thinks they are broken because they sneezed.

But why is it that I don't feel shame about my burst appendix, but I do feel shame about my panic attacks? When the body is hurt—when there's disease, a broken bone, an open wound or a burn—it isn't considered a personal failure of the individual. But depression, anxiety, mood disorders and personality disorders are more usually seen as states for which the individual who is suffering is personally responsible, and the society in which we live seems to cultivate the delusion that it holds no responsibility for such things. What if my panic attacks aren't actually a sign of personal failure or an indicator that I can't cope with life? What if they're more systemic—an indicator that the world in which we live is not an easy place to be?

Our emotions don't live in the same temporal world that our bodies do. There is another entire geography within ourselves that I would argue has nothing to do with our working selves or even our consuming selves. Our internal, emotional lives are complex, contradictory, irrational and extremely powerful. The half-life of a seemingly trivial event from childhood can last decades. I believe that if we want to explore our emotional landscapes, it helps to have the guidance of a mental health professional. A few sessions with a psychologist will punch some sizeable holes in any adult's belief that by simply moving forward in time they have magically become a different person from who they were at eight, or eighteen. It's a strange but enlightening process to learn more about your psychological self.

But not many people can afford to spend $100, $200, or even $300 an hour on a psychologist. Psychotherapy is still a privilege of the middle classes. I've been lucky in my life to have had access to subsidised therapy several times, and when I couldn't get that I decided to spend the money anyway. I gave up having a decent car, taking holidays or contributing to my super or my savings. Over the years, the money I have spent on therapy would probably add up to a deposit for a house. I don't regret it, but I know that many people can't afford such support on top of their day-to-day expenses, and instead are on long waiting lists for free or more affordable counselling.

Access to therapy isn't a silver bullet for anxiety disorders. For me, though, therapy has given me detailed knowledge of myself, of my emotional geography. This knowledge has gone a long way in helping me when those highly charged states of irrational panic hit me. It has helped me to understand that I am not my panic, that I am so much more than the storm I am currently passing through.

Last year, I moved from Australia to New Zealand. Along with my container-load of belongings, I also found room for my anxiety, as if I had brought a special gold suitcase labelled 'To Be Opened in Emergencies (Or Any Old Time Really).' Moving countries shook up my entire identity and things have not quite settled. I have not quite settled.

My wife and I live outside of the city, so our surroundings are quiet—maybe a little too quiet. I have views of hills and rivers instead of skyscrapers, and the afternoon rush hour consists of a mob of wild turkeys moving across the house paddock. But the geography of my inner world remains the same. It's a complex terrain that still has its share of difficult weather, but the more I understand this place, the better chance I have of withstanding the storms when they arise.

A Short History of Unease

D.A. Glynn

There was a time, if you'd asked me what I was anxious about, I might have answered, *pace* Brando, 'Whaddaya got?' Except I wasn't that cool, and no one ever asked.

They didn't need to. It was generally acknowledged that I was a 'sensitive' child, and anxiety was just a subset of that sensitivity. Yet, looking back, it seems to me that for much of my childhood and adolescence what I really was was anxious, about everything, all of the time.

Where it began, who could say? I remember being a tear-stained five-year-old, stalled at the gates of Torbay Primary on my first day of school, my mother pulling me one way and me pulling the other. But I doubt that was the true beginning. Most likely it was there from the outset—latent, atavistic—a tiny homunculus clinging at the base of my brain.

In Rollo May's comprehensive study, *The Meaning of Anxiety*, published in 1950, he notes that anxiety can be observed in infants in just the second week of life. So probably it's in all of us, one way or another, and some more than others. A five-year-old not wanting to go to school is unremarkable. If by this time they are also scared of the dark, well, that's hardly unusual, either.

For May, the question of anxiety is how it is differentiated from fear. At the age of six, my own personality was scarcely formed, and if my anxieties about going to school had not yet been provided a particular object to fix upon, that oversight was about to be rectified.

Hobyahs.

Let me tell you the story as I remember it. A little girl lives in a cottage with an old man and an old woman and a little dog. The hobyahs, for whom no real description is provided, live out in the cane. Their stated intention, whispered amongst themselves, is to enter the house, eat the old man and the old woman, put the little girl in a sack and make off with her, to eat her at their leisure.

The first night the hobyahs come out of the cane toward the house, the little dog barks, scaring them away. Next morning the old man, annoyed by the dog's barking, decides the best course of action is to cut off one of the dog's legs. The hobyahs return the next night, and the next night, and the next, with similar outcome. Unfortunately, by then the little dog has run out of legs to cut off, so the old man makes do with its head.

No more barking. The hobyahs return again, this time making good on their intent. The old man and old woman are eaten, the little girl carried off in a sack.

I don't know if I'd stopped listening by then, or maybe entered into some kind of fugue state. I have since discovered, looking up the story on the internet, that it had some sort of happy ending—a passing hunter with a large dog kills the hobyahs and rescues the little girl. Back then, all I knew was that if the night had not previously contained any specific fears, it sure as hell did now.

Freud, in his *Introductory Lectures on Psycho-analysis*, wrote that 'one thing is certain, that the problem of anxiety is a nodal point, linking up all kinds of most important questions; a riddle, of which the solution must cast a flood of light upon our whole mental life.'[1] Note that for Freud the problem is 'anxiety', not 'fear'. With the rise of the psychological professions in the 20th century, the question of whether fear led to anxiety or vice

---

1 Sigmund Freud, *Introductory Lectures on Psycho-Analysis* (London, UK: Hogarth Press, 1956–1974), 393.

versa was much discussed. Fear was assumed to be the generic state and anxiety its derivative. Yet, developmentally, it seemed plain that fear follows from anxiety.

One thing that was agreed was that 'anxiety is to be distinguished from fear in that fear has a specific object, whereas anxiety is a vague and unspecific apprehension.'[2] Fear is objective, anxiety subjective. In various languages the correct form is, generally, 'I have a fear' but 'I am anxious'. You could say that anxiety is the highway we travel, with various attractions—unease, nervousness, dread, fear, panic—to keep us entertained along the way.

So, *was* I afraid of hobyahs, specifically? Not necessarily—I think that even aged six I could differentiate between real and imaginary beings. By far the more disturbing part of the tale, to me, was the old man's treatment of the little dog. Probably what ratcheted my anxiety up another notch was the idea that random things, for which you had no defence, could just happen. Little dogs could get their legs cut off. (He was only trying to help!) Worse, teachers at school could tell you stories about it and you had no choice but to listen. I mean, it was like they were *trying* to disturb you, something with which I didn't need any help.

From that point my memory becomes clearer, and my anxieties become more my own. One holiday, at most a year or two later, my family and I stayed in a bach in Whitianga. As I lay in an unfamiliar bed on what was probably a Saturday night, I could hear a vague commotion of voices, distant and indistinct. I don't know how long it took me to work it out, but at some point I realised the cause: plainly it was an escaped lion, who was pursuing the people of Whitianga noisily along the town's main street, ever closer to where I lay.

Interestingly, I just lay there, this scenario playing in my

---

2   Rollo May, *The Meaning of Anxiety* (New York: Ronald Press, 1950), 51.

head. Maybe it was that the commotion never seemed to get any closer, or maybe it was because I knew that the idea was too outlandish to be taken seriously. Eventually I fell asleep. The following morning, someone asked if we'd been kept awake by the party going on next door. Well, no—I was kept awake by an escaped lion.

I never mentioned that incident, though I still remember it vividly four and a half decades later. I don't remember voicing my anxieties, increasing as they were both in quality and quantity, to anyone.

Probably my anxiety was the reason I got so many headaches. They were diagnosed as migraines, though they weren't ascribed to any specific physical cause. They just came, with depressing regularity. But they had their uses.

At school it was decided—possibly by the same authority who thought that reading us a story about murderous hobyahs and dog-maiming old men was a good idea—that skipping would be an ideal form of physical exercise, the kind with one long rope and one hapless individual in the middle, their performance plain for all to see.

At that stage I was singularly uncoordinated, so suddenly there was another thing to be anxious about. But if anxiety was going to give me headaches, I could use those headaches to negate one source of anxiety, at least. Whether my teachers ever noticed the regularity of those migraines, which every week came on in the hour before skipping practice, they certainly never pressed the issue, and I was spared the problem of facing . . . whatever it was I so didn't want to face.

Not skipping, per se—I wasn't anxious about falling over and breaking my nose. There is a difference between what we might think of as objective (or 'normal') anxiety and neurotic anxiety. Objective anxiety is the natural reaction to an external danger, and is both rational and useful. The development of anxiety disproportionate to the amount of danger, or where no ostensible danger exists, is neurotic anxiety. So I guess I was anxious about the embarrassment of falling over in public, not any pain or injury that might occur.

Freud, with reasoning which might at first glance seem circular, deemed anxiety 'the fundamental phenomenon and the central problem of neurosis'.[3] This seems reasonable. Then again, Freud generally ascribed the origin of anxiety to birth trauma and a fear of castration. So there's that.

I don't know how much birth trauma or fear of castration I might have had—I'm thinking not very much. But I do know that as a child I was anxious about a whole raft of things, none of which presented any actual danger: anxious about going to school camp, about having to speak in front of the class, about being crap at football, and so on.

Was I neurotic? I don't know. I functioned more than adequately and as mentioned above, no one ever asked what I was so worried about, nor did I feel the need to voice my apprehensions. I mean, I *knew* that being afraid of going to school camp was stupid. But anxiety is the shadow of intellect, as someone once said, and if I was uncoordinated, shy and fearful, I was also a thinker, even then, and I guess that's just the price I paid.

Eventually, I stopped being scared of the dark. I went to school camp and it turned out to be fun. I gave up playing football. The migraines abated. Then arose the problem of girls.

Modesty prevents me detailing all of my anxieties when it came to sex and relationships, save to say they were many and varied. Thankfully, it turns out, they were largely unfounded.

---

[3] Sigmund Freud, *The Problem of Anxiety* (New York: Psychoanalytic Quarterly Press and W.W. Norton, 1936), 85.

Would that I'd known that at the time.

If we can discount Freud's literal notions—no one is actually traumatised by being born, nor do genitals lie at the root of all psychological problems—they still retain some symbolic value. Psychologists later came to view anxiety as a problem of individuation, a process of which separation from the mother at birth is just the first stage. Otto Rank saw a person's life history as being an endless series of separations, with each experience presenting the possibility of a greater autonomy for the individual. What he characterised as 'life fear' is the anxiety that occurs at every new possibility of autonomous activity, or 'the fear of having to live as an isolated individual.'[4] So we are obliged to negotiate these ongoing separations, internally, in the process of becoming ourselves. Then we must renegotiate them, externally, in the process of forming relationships with the world.

If for me that problem resolved itself eventually, it was not without a few years of unnecessary torment. As a teenager, the task of integrating myself and then reintegrating with the world was challenging enough, without the added impediment of having no real knowledge about girls. Much of the time it felt easier to just give up. I mean, there was always television.

Most days after school I would come home, fix myself something to eat—cornflakes, toast and peanut butter—then lie on the floor in front of the TV, watch *M*A*S*H* or *Happy Days* or whatever was on, until six o'clock, which was dinner time.

Invariably, at around 5:30, I would hear my father's wagon arrive in the carport below. My father was a carpet-layer. It was hard work, but two minutes after I'd heard him arrive he would literally bound up the stairs, so happy was he to be home. (It was a spiral staircase, with wooden treads, and my father was

---

[4] Otto Rank, *Will Therapy: An Analysis of the Therapeutic Process in Terms of Relationship* (New York: Alfred A. Knopf, 1936), 175.

a big man, so the whole assembly vibrated under his feet; I'll never forget the sound it made.) Then one day I noticed that he no longer ran up the stairs. He only walked.

I don't know how long it took. Months, maybe. And no one ever said anything. He just got slower and slower, until eventually he could barely crawl up those stairs, dragging himself with his hands. Meanwhile, I lay on the floor, trying and failing to concentrate on the TV. I didn't know what the hell was happening to my dad, but I sure as hell knew it wasn't good.

It was kidney stones. My brother and I were away surfing the weekend he passed the largest of them—fortunately, my mother told us; it meant we weren't there to hear him scream. He was a brave man: when he was 21 he'd cut off half of his thumb on a table saw, so he knew pain, but that kidney stone was a mass of jagged shards of calcium, and I don't even want to imagine what it must have felt like coming out. One of his kidneys was ruined and then the other went out in sympathy, and if you don't have your kidneys, well, pretty soon you're going, too.

Of all the separations a person has to face, death is the ultimate one. In philosophical terms, anxiety can be described as a person's reaction to the threat of a concept called nonbeing. But as Rollo May writes in *The Meaning of Anxiety*, 'the threat of nonbeing lies in the psychological and spiritual realms as well, namely the threat of meaninglessness in one's existence.'[5] And it's not hard to see how the two notions—nonbeing and meaninglessness—might intertwine in the mind of a sensitive teenager, and bring anxiety to a whole new level.

'When he woke up in the morning everything was white, and he knew that today was the day his father was going to die.'

5 May, 12.

I wrote that sentence some time between the ages of 16 and 25, I think. Where I grew up, in Auckland in the 1970s, winter still brought the occasional hard frost, and I believe I did look out of my bedroom window one morning to see that everything was white.

I don't recall what I had in mind, whether it was the beginning of a short story or even a novel. I do know that the 'I' wasn't actually me, and that if anything followed on from that sentence it is long since lost. But those exact words I have never forgotten. As it was, my father didn't die on that day. He was given a kidney transplant, and lived in comparatively good health for about a decade.[6] If I was adjusted to the situation, it may have been because death no longer seemed imminent. I know that generally my various anxieties had diminished over time, and perhaps that was because, in light of that meta-anxiety, they had come to assume a more proper proportion.

In 1844 Søren Kierkegaard published *The Concept of Anxiety*, which was the first philosophical treatment of what he termed *angst*, originally translated as 'dread'. Kierkegaard's fundamental insight was to bind the concept of anxiety to that of freedom. He defines freedom as 'possibility'. Rollo May summarises it this way: 'Kierkegaard sees man as the creature who is continually beckoned by possibility, who conceives of possibility, visualizes it, and by creative activity carries it into actuality.'[7] Anxiety, for Kierkegaard, is the state that individuals feel when they confront this freedom, this possibility. What is required then is an act of creativity in order to transform possibility into reality. The more possibility an individual has, the more potential anxiety they'll experience at the same time.

The problem—the source, as it were—of anxiety is that

---

6   My father died at the (not quite) ripe old age of 60, and honesty compels me to note that his death troubled me more than perhaps it should have. But that's another essay.

7   May, 32.

people, bound by death, are finite, and we know it. Yet within those bounds we are free. The theologian Reinhold Niebuhr sums it up like this: 'In short, man, being both bound and free, both limited and limitless, is anxious. Anxiety is the inevitable concomitant of the paradox of freedom and finiteness in which man is involved.'[8]

What's interesting to me is how we seem to know this, even as infants and certainly as children. How it is the struggle against anxiety, through the creative act—creating both ourselves and the artefacts of our lives—which dictates the person we become. And if it takes the possibility of death to force one to write a sentence, just as it takes the possibility of life to force one to live, then isn't it better than to embrace that and to prosper? Kierkegaard again: 'I would say that learning to know anxiety is an adventure which every man has to affront if he would not go to perdition either by not having known anxiety or by sinking under it. He therefore who has learned rightly to be anxious has learned the most important thing.'

I don't know how much I actually learned. Over time—it was decades, probably—I stopped being anxious almost entirely. And rather than learn to write, I think I shed all of those things which had stopped from writing successfully. It all seemed to happen quite naturally. But there is a lesson, and if I could go back and talk to myself when I was seven, I'd tell him, 'At some point, kid, you're going to have to skip.'

---

[8] Reinhold Niebuhr, *The Nature and Destiny of Man* (New York, NY: C. Scribner's Sons, 1941), 182.

Micronutrients and Mental Health

An interview with Meredith Blampied and Julia Rucklidge

In 2011–2012, Te Rau Hinengaro: The New Zealand Mental Health Survey found that 15 percent of all adults surveyed had experienced an anxiety disorder in the past 12 months—higher than depression and substance abuse combined. At the University of Canterbury's Mental Health and Nutrition Laboratory, clinical psychologists Meredith Blampied and Professor Julia Rucklidge are investigating the role of micronutrients in mental health, including for people suffering post-earthquake trauma. Here, they outline the state of anxiety healthcare in New Zealand and suggest an alternative based on their clinical trials.
—Naomi Arnold

NA: *What is anxiety? Why do we get it?*
MB and JR: We are all hauntingly familiar with that sensation—the dropping of the gut, the rash of goosebumps across the body, the sudden leap of the heart. Some of us might feel flushed, others cold. Some start to shake, and others find themselves stiff and frozen. Usually the mind starts to race, but sometimes it goes blank. All of these are features of the threat response, one of the oldest responses in the human body. The threat response is not a uniquely human feature. It is shared across many of our animal cousins. We can easily identify a threatened dog, a scared cat, a possum frozen in the centre of the road. Often referred to as the fight/flight/freeze/flop reaction, it aims to keeps us safe from harm, vigilant to potential threat and able to protect others. As a cornerstone of our survival, it

is unsurprising this threat response plays an important role in our mental health.

Anxiety is closely associated with the threat response, adapting and modifying it in relation to the situations with which we are faced. We don't all immediately escalate to full-blown panic. Sometimes we can spend days with a low-level sense of dread and anticipation. Our brains, the infinitely complex organs that they are, have learned to temper and measure this response to find the most appropriate survival option. Some situations call for a speedy retreat. Some call for careful consideration and planning. And some life-threatening situations require anger and self-defence.

To ensure our survival, the brain attempts to understand the situation, our goals and our values to decide on the safest outcome for us and our families; however, the brain does not always make the best choices. Some of us have huge difficulty managing the threat response and, subsequently, managing our anxiety. Genetics and early life experiences may play a role, causing excessive levels of anxiety in situations that objectively don't call for such a response. Perhaps one of our parents was anxious, and, from an early age, we observed this significant person modelling anxious responses to possibly non-threatening situations. This can inadvertently teach us to respond in the same way. Maybe we have been through traumatic and dangerous situations that have sensitised our bodies and brains to be hyper-vigilant to danger at all times, on the constant lookout to keep us safe. Some scientists also point to modern society: high stress levels, financial difficulties, social media overuse and reduced social support can heighten our anxiety response to a state beyond what is reasonable or optimal.[1]

That 15 percent of adults over the past year here in New

---

1 See, for example, N. Smyth et al., 'Social Networks, Social Support and Psychiatric Symptoms', *Social Psychiatry and Psychiatric Epidemiology* 50, no. 7 (2015): 1111–120.

Zealand have experienced moderate or seriously impairing anxiety disorders is very concerning. This survey did not capture those people experiencing anxiety who did not meet criteria for a diagnosis. Research has indicated that these 'sub-threshold' conditions can also place a costly burden on individuals and society more widely.[2]

What are the treatment options and how effective are they?
Fortunately, anxiety and its related disorders are among the most treatable health conditions. Treatment follows a 'stepped care' model based on symptom severity. Generally, lower intensity treatment options (education, e-therapy, self-help) are successful for treating less severe anxiety problems. Psychological therapy is usually recommended as the next step of care, followed by psychiatric medication as a stand-alone treatment or as an adjunct to psychological therapy.

It is difficult to measure the efficacy of stepped care models, as they are often implemented in varied ways, taking into account different healthcare systems. However, evidence generally suggests that, for anxiety, stepped care models can provide an effective method of rationing and guiding appropriate treatment.[3]

We often hear that people struggle to access psychological treatment, whether privately (because of cost) or through the New Zealand health system (because of availability).
Yes, in New Zealand we face a shortage of accessible and available treatment options for anxiety disorders. There is a

---

[2] See, for example, D. Berardi et al., 'Mental, Physical and Functional Status in Primary Care Attenders', *International Journal of Psychiatry in Medicine* 29, no. 2 (1999): 133–48.

[3] See, for example, F.Y.-Y. Ho et al., 'The Efficacy and Cost-Effectiveness of Stepped Care Prevention and Treatment for Depressive and/or Anxiety Disorders', *Scientific Reports* 6 (2016): 29281.

nationwide shortage of clinical psychologists and psychiatrists, which means that jobs remain vacant and many people do not have access to appropriate professionals who can provide treatment. Publicly funded psychological therapy or psychiatric intervention is also limited, and there is only one publicly funded tertiary treatment service specifically devoted to the treatment of anxiety disorders (this is in Canterbury). These treatment options are insufficient, given the number of people who need specialised anxiety treatment. Evidence also suggests that psychologists with high competence in the treatment of specific anxiety difficulties have improved treatment outcomes.[4]

We shouldn't forget that, although psychological treatments for anxiety are effective at improving symptoms without the danger of adverse side effects, there are still a number of people who receive psychological treatment for anxiety and continue to struggle with their symptoms, making a partial or limited recovery.

What other factors influence the recovery process?
If you are unable to attend therapy appointments, you are less likely to recover. If you are unable to find or choose a therapist who suits your needs (a common phenomenon in a public healthcare system with limited staff), you may be less likely to improve. If you don't have enough time in your day-to-day life to reflect on your therapy or practise the skills you have learned, you are less likely to overcome your anxiety difficulties.

With all these potential obstacles, it is unsurprising that up to 30 percent of individuals may discontinue therapy, 30–40 percent may report little or no change and 5–15 percent of people may report negative effects as a consequence of therapy. From a practical perspective, if there are no competent and

---

4   See, for example, D.M. Ginzburg et al., 'Treatment Specific Competence Predicts Outcome in Cognitive Therapy for Social Anxiety Disorder', *Behaviour Research and Therapy* 50, no. 12 (2012): 747–52.

experienced anxiety-focussed psychologists available to treat you at a price you can afford, you are unlikely to be able to receive psychological treatment.

There are a lot of online resources and apps, like Calm and Headspace. How good are these at helping people with anxiety?
Unfortunately, despite these services being easily accessible, uptake is poor, perhaps due to difficulties accessing the internet or lack of support completing the various therapy modules. Indeed, research demonstrates that although self-help and e-therapies are effective, motivation and therapist contact can impact on whether or not symptoms improve.[5]

Prescriptions for psychiatric medications such as SSRIs have been on the rise in New Zealand. Are these being used in place of psychological treatment?
The high rate of prescriptions may be a consequence of publicly funded medication, ease of access through GPs, and limited access to other forms of treatment, such as psychotherapy.

Although medications such as anxiolytics are not identified by treatment guidelines as the first line of treatment for anxiety disorders, Pharmac statistics indicate that medications including SSRIs and anxiolytics are being used more frequently to treat these disorders in New Zealand. Prescribing rates for antidepressants (also used for the treatment of anxiety disorders) increased 5 percent between 2015 and 2017, by a total of approximately 70,000 prescriptions. There has been a 22 percent increase in the scripting of antidepressants over the past five years, and, according to Pharmac publication *Going to Your Head*, in 2016 alone a total of 1.6 million scripts for antidepressant medications were written.

5   See, for example, M.G. Newman et al., 'A Review of Technology-Assisted Self-Help and Minimal Contact Therapies for Anxiety and Depression', *Clinical Psychology Review* 31, no. 1 (2011) 89–103.

How effective are they?
While these medications have been demonstrated as effective in improving anxiety symptoms, too many people do not achieve full relief from medications. This can be due to difficulty tolerating the side effects that are common with anxiety medications, but it can also be the result of continuing to experience functionally impairing symptoms despite several medication trials. Medications for anxiety difficulties have a range of well-known adverse side effects, including loss of sexual interest, weight changes, physical agitation and feeling emotionally numb. For some, the medications simply do not provide the expected relief from symptoms. So despite access to a number of different evidence-based treatments, not enough people are experiencing full relief from their symptoms.

You've been gathering evidence for nutrition as an alternative approach to treating anxiety. Can you tell us about your research? How much evidence is there that nutritional interventions are an effective way forward?
Current medical models of mental health view distress and emotional instability as an illness in the brain, to be treated by intervening and changing brain functioning. However, this approach misses the link between the brain and its place in our body as an organ that is intrinsically linked to other bodily functions. The importance of diet and nutrition in physical health is conclusive, and it is well understood that maintaining a healthy diet can prevent heart disease, cancer, diabetes and other poor health outcomes. The field of mental health has lagged behind in the integration of diet into treatment of emotional distress, perhaps due to the predominant medical model being used as a guiding treatment modality. Over the past decade, a number of dedicated researchers have started to explore the link between nutrition and mental health.

Research investigating the impact of diet on brain function

in our animal cousins has found that high-fat, high-sugar diets and irregular eating patterns were associated with increased anxiety in rats. The same study also found that poor maternal nutrition resulted in offspring with higher anxiety.[6]

What about tests of human subjects?
For ethical reasons, testing the same dietary manipulations in humans has been more difficult. Nevertheless, observational studies have demonstrated that the diet of individuals experiencing mental health issues are routinely more nutritionally deprived than those without the same issues. Chronic life stress has also been associated with a greater intake of high-fat, high-sugar diets.

So is a poor diet causing the anxiety, or is the anxiety causing a poor diet? What should someone with anxiety eat if they hope to improve symptoms?
Of all the different diets of societies, the Mediterranean diet has been found to convey positive mental and physical health benefits. Characterised by high consumption of vegetables, nuts, grains, olive oil and a moderate amount of protein, a recent well-designed study found this diet improved depressive symptoms for participants.[7] These results are promising and deserve more focus and attention.

But if you struggle with anxiety or depression, it's extra difficult to find the energy, time and inclination to eat well.
Many of us know the difficulties in making long-term, sustainable changes to our diet, especially if we're also

6   See M. Murphy and J.G. Mercer, 'Diet-Regulated Anxiety', *International Journal of Endocrinology* 2013 (2013) and S. Dutheil et al., 'High-Fat Diet Induced Anxiety and Anhedonia', *Neuropsychopharmacology* 41, no. 7 (2016): 1874.

7   F.N. Jacka et al., 'A Randomised Controlled Trial of Dietary Improvement for Adults with Major Depression', *BMC Medicine* 15, no. 1 (2017): 23.

struggling to manage our mental health. Our research asks: is there a role for nutritional supplementation in improving our anxiety, perhaps by taking a pill of a different nature?

What kind of nutrients are we talking about?
A range of research studies have explored the role of individual nutrients in improving anxiety. The B vitamin group has demonstrable positive effects, as have omega-3 and magnesium. This again is promising work, although a review indicated some variability in the data—small to moderate effects and difficulties replicating the same positive effects in subsequent studies. It may be that nutrients taken in isolation are not the answer to improving anxiety. The body is a marvellously complicated place and, given this, it is unsurprising that it may require a more complex nutrient approach.

Emerging evidence suggests that improving anxiety may come down to providing the broad spectrum of vitamins and minerals in combination in order to provide the body with the nutrients it needs for optimal brain function. It is unclear at this stage whether this approach is correcting nutritional deficiencies or, perhaps more likely, correcting deficiencies *relative to that individual's metabolic needs*. Micronutrients give the body a wide range of all the vitamins and minerals necessary for functioning, in doses and forms that survive being broken down by stomach acid and can compensate for poor gut absorption. It seems that this combined nutrient approach using micronutrients may be more effective than the single nutrient approach that has predominated the research literature for the past one hundred years.

What has your research shown so far?
Micronutrients have been demonstrated as effective at helping adults and children with symptoms associated with ADHD to reduce stress and improve resilience following a range of natural

disasters. Micronutrients also appear effective at improving insomnia, stress and anxiety in adults presenting for treatment of sleep difficulties. Several additional studies have also demonstrated that, compared with placebos, micronutrients collectively can help improve stress in healthy adults.[8]

How do they work?
Many possible pathways have been suggested to explain how micronutrients might improve mental health. Perhaps micronutrients improve our gut's ability to absorb nutrients? It is also possible that they assist pathways in the brain to function more effectively and improve our mitochondrial and membrane functioning. Inflammation has recently been implicated in poor mental health, and it's possible that micronutrients reduce inflammation caused by oxidative stress or immune reactions. Micronutrients may also help us compensate for genetic errors that impact our ability to metabolise nutrients effectively. Perhaps they simply replenish the body of nutrients after years of supporting an overactive fight-or-flight response. All these possible explanations would suggest that to effectively treat mental health conditions, including anxiety, broad-spectrum micronutrient interventions are needed.

What about safety?
A 2011 review of micronutrient treatment explored biological safety data from 144 adults and children, and found no clinically meaningful negative outcomes and no serious adverse events linked to the micronutrient formula.[9] Since then, further

---

[8] See, for example, S.J. Long and D. Benton, 'Effects of Vitamin and Mineral Supplementation on Stress, Mild Psychiatric Symptoms, and Mood in Nonclinical Samples: A Meta-Analysis', *Psychosomatic Medicine* 75, no. 2 (2013): 144–53.

[9] J.S.A. Simpson et al., 'Systematic Review of Safety and Tolerability of a Complex Micronutrient Formula Used in Mental Health', *BMC Psychiatry* 11, no. 1 (2011): 62.

safety outcome data on micronutrient intervention has found similar results. In two randomised controlled trials comparing micronutrients with placebos, there were no group differences in side effects. This means that those taking micronutrients reported as many side effects as those taking placebos. This is good news. And what are the most common side effects reported from taking capsules? Headaches and nausea.[10] More promising is that these symptoms dissipate within a few weeks and by ensuring the capsules are taken with food and water.

The onus continues to fall on researchers to firmly establish the safety and tolerability of micronutrients, and ongoing research continues to collect, measure and interpret safety-related data from trials; however, when the side effects are compared with the commonly accepted side-effect profiles of anxiety medications, micronutrients appear to be the intervention with the fewest adverse side effects. With continued trials exploring the efficacy and effectiveness of micronutrients in treating anxiety difficulties specifically, the current research picture seems promising.

If micronutrient supplementation is so effective, why aren't doctors prescribing or recommending this treatment as a first option?
The area of nutrition and mental health is a relatively new field and has yet to be conclusively demonstrated as effective for widespread treatment of mental health issues. It is important to establish effectiveness prior to healthcare professionals recommending these treatments to people, outside of clinical trials. However, as more evidence is collected about the positive effect of micronutrients, this is changing. Ultimately, there is a treatment gap in New Zealand for people with anxiety who need to access responsive, effective, appropriate and safe treatment.

10 J.J. Rucklidge et al., 'Vitamin–Mineral Treatment of Attention-Deficit Hyperactivity Disorder in Adults', *British Journal of Psychiatry* 204, no. 4 (2014): 306–15.

A micronutrient approach to anxiety difficulties may be one solution to filling this gap in the New Zealand stepped care model of treatment. As we continue to explore the effectiveness and safety of these interventions, a picture begins to emerge. It may be possible that, in the next five years, you are offered a micronutrient approach when asking your primary-care provider for help with anxiety.

To change a well-established healthcare approach is difficult. If we want to establish micronutrients as a healthcare approach, then information about micronutrients and their impact on anxiety would need to be disseminated at the highest level, with policymakers and funding bodies actively involved. The same information would need to be available to hard-working practitioners and to people who struggle with anxiety. Perhaps one day micronutrients will have a place in the existing stepped care model for anxiety in Aotearoa.

No one treatment solves everything; micronutrients won't solve all of our woes, conflicts and worries about the future. We might still experience that gut-dropping sensation and the prickle of goosebumps up our arms. But micronutrients might provide a safe and effective first line of treatment for some people needing help with their anxiety.

For more information on Meredith Blampied and Julia Rucklidge's research, visit Mental Health and Nutrition Research Group at canterbury.ac.nz

Further reading

H.C. Woods and H. Scott, '#SleepyTeens: Social Media Use in Adolescence is Associated with Poor Sleep Quality, Anxiety, Depression and Low Self-Esteem', *Journal of Adolescence* 51 (2016): 41–49.

C.-W et al., 'Managing Stress and Anxiety through Qigong Exercise in Healthy Adults', *BMC Complementary and Alternative Medicine* 14, no. 1 (2014): 8.

J.M. Newby et al., 'Systematic Review and Meta-Analysis of Trans-diagnostic Psychological Treatments for Anxiety and Depressive Disorders in Adulthood', *Clinical Psychology Review* 40 (2015): 91–110.

T. Nordgreen et al., 'Stepped Care Versus Direct Face-to-Face Cognitive Behavior Therapy for Social Anxiety Disorder and Panic Disorder', *Behavior Therapy* 47 no. 2 (2016): 166–83.

G. Burlingame et al., *Bergin and Garfield's Handbook of Psychotherapy and Behavior Change* (New York, NY: Wiley, 2004).

S.J. Torres and C.A. Nowson, 'Relationship Between Stress, Eating Behavior, and Obesity', *Nutrition* 23, no. 11 (2007): 887–94.

C. Davis et al., 'Definition of the Mediterranean Diet: A Literature Review', *Nutrients* 7, no. 11 (2015): 9139–153.

Hibbeln, J.R., *Depression, Suicide and Deficiencies of Omega-3 Essential Fatty Acids in Modern Diets*, in *Omega-3 Fatty Acids, the Brain and Retina* (Karger Publishers, 2009), 17–30.

B.J. Kaplan et al., 'A Randomised Trial of Nutrient Supplements to Minimise Psychological Stress after a Natural Disaster', *Psychiatry Research* 228, no. 3 (2015): 373–79.

J.J. Rucklidge et al., 'Shaken but Unstirred? Effects of Micronutrients on Stress and Trauma after an Earthquake', *Human Psychopharmacology: Clinical and Experimental* 27, no. 5 (2012): 440–54.

J. Lothian, N.M. Blampied and J.J. Rucklidge, 'Effect of Micronutrients on Insomnia in Adults: A Multiple-Baseline Study', *Clinical Psychological Science* 4, no. 6 (2016): 1112–124.

B.J. Kaplan et al., 'The Emerging Field of Nutritional Mental Health: Inflammation, the Microbiome, Oxidative Stress, and Mitochondrial Function', *Clinical Psychological Science* 3, no. 6 (2015): 964–80.

Ghost Knife

Ashleigh Young

The truth is dark under your eyelids.
What are you going to do about it?
—Charles Simic[1]

Most nights before I fall asleep, and sometimes during a quiet moment in the day, I can feel a knife floating above my right shoulder. It's a distinctive knife, with a broad blade and a generous handle. A good knife for cutting up a pumpkin. Still, for a sharp, pointy object, it's nebulous; I can't tell exactly what shape it is. As it floats meditatively I feel a slight pressure. Then the knife begins to stab the side of my face. It focusses on my right side, burying itself in the little hollow below my cheekbone and moving across to my jaw, making short, but deep, strokes along the way. Occasionally the knife makes these incisions with care, as if getting started on a surgical procedure; other times the work is rapid and violent. And sometimes the knife shape-shifts into another pointed object, like a pair of chopsticks, or a long skewer, the sort that you'd use to test whether a leg of lamb was cooked through. It's even been the little triangular wedge I put under my front door to stop the wind from slamming it shut.

'Because the right side of the body is governed by the left side of the brain,' an alternative healer tells me, 'it could be that this imagined stabbing is to do with some avoidance or procrastination in your life.' The healer, who is massaging my

1 'Against Winter', *New and Selected Poems 1962–2012* (New York, NY: Houghton Mifflin Harcourt, 2013), 217.

head and face as I lie on a table, continues, 'So it may be, simply, that you need to do your chores.' Then he draws a card for me from his tarot deck, and it's the salmon. The wisest animal! The salmon is swimming upriver in search of a spawning ground, leaping over obstacles in its rush to get there. But somehow, according to the tarot cards, it's also possible that I'm the opposite of the salmon. The silliest animal, recklessly swimming downstream.

Although the knife is not something I can truly see or feel, the thought of it creates an abstract pressure that spreads across my cheek and into my ear, so I often feel tense there, and have the sense that I shouldn't make sudden movements. The head massage softens some of this pressure, at least. I pay the guy and go back to work, where I write a to-do list and do the first few things on it. But that night the knife is hanging around my head as usual, just as it has for the past year.

I've never literally stabbed myself in the face; at least not on purpose. When I was a toddler I cut open one side of my mouth on the sharp metal edge of a chair and, a few days later, the *other* side of my mouth on the *exact same chair*, so that I had facial wounds like the Joker's, but that's about it. One of the reasons I'm agitated by the knife is that it's so at odds with the version of myself I recognise. If there are 'knife people', I'm not one of them. I'm not even a very violent person! I sometimes ignite with rage when I'm riding my bike; once I rode at full speed—like the salmon, leaping upriver—in pursuit of a truck that had nudged me into the gutter, and when I caught up with it I pounded on its window and screamed, while the driver shrugged. But you have to believe me that that was a contained incident.

My ghost knife can probably be defined as an intrusive thought—an unwanted and unpleasant thought that pops up from time to time. Intrusive thoughts are near universal. They might feel unwholesome and seem to cast doubt on your moral character or even your sanity, but you don't have to be suffering from any clinical condition to experience them. It's intrusive to think of standing up in the middle of a formal meeting and shouting 'Balls!' before overturning the table, but the thought doesn't mean you'll go through with it. You probably won't slap the head of the person sitting in front of you on the bus, or do a backflip at a funeral, even if for a second you have the strong conviction that you're about to do so. I think most of us have the conscience and impulse control to stop us from carrying out acts like that. When approaching a table on a street outside a cafe, I might fear that I'm about to grab a handful of hot chips off a stranger's plate and stuff them in my mouth while sprinting off, but then I'll find myself walking past with my hands in my pockets.

There are also those intrusive thoughts that are simply distressing mental images and not necessarily to do with the deliberate violation of a social norm. You might picture a person being run over by a bus, or imagine a shark barrelling towards you when you dive into a public pool. The images can visit in a single flash behind your eyes or play out before you as a detailed scene.

Sometimes when I'm arriving home at the end of the day, tired from riding my bike uphill, I am sure, sickeningly sure, that I'm about to see my cat's body on the road. I brace myself as I cruise down the pathway to the letterbox, knowing that my mental image of a small white furry body in the gutter is about to come true. The fact that it doesn't come true and that every day my cat Jerry canters down the steps after me and into the house does not keep me from experiencing the same thought at the same time the next day, and I can almost feel the thought etching its shape permanently into my mind, like my first phone number or my own middle name.

Conventional psychiatric wisdom, and plenty of religious interpretation, says that such thoughts are involuntary: a minor misfiring in the brain rather than a reflection of who you are. The wisdom says that there is a definitive you, a core identity, and these thoughts come from not-you—a threatening outside entity that's trying to make you come undone. 'I call her Ollie,' writes one mental health blogger. 'She's the one whispering the intrusive thoughts to me.' The wisdom insists that if a sinister thought is frequent, it might point to some underlying problem, but it doesn't mean that at heart you're bad or unhinged.

I can believe this utterly of other people and their thoughts. But when it comes to my knife, I'm not convinced. Surely the knife means I'm at least slightly evil or slightly crazy. Where has it come from, if not my own subconscious? Is it trying to warn me of something, like a dog that's trained to sniff out cancerous tumors? And why does it stab that specific spot on my face? Perhaps unsurprisingly, the knife often comes when I'm thinking of the things I've promised to do but haven't yet, or wondering how I will explain that I can't meet a deadline, or remembering how a talk I gave went badly. These thoughts are the knife's siren song.

Even if I'm right that the knife springs from guilt and self-loathing, I don't understand which part of my *self* it is trying to harm—if the self can be broken into constituent parts. Is it my physical self? Emotional, intellectual, neurological? Which part of me does it want to harm most, or does it have a general aversion to my existence altogether? Sometimes, in defence, I try to imagine myself as without solid form, like a pile of blossom, and when the knife plunges into me it scatters me to the wind.

When I was a kid I read a story in the *New Zealand School Journal* about a herd of cows that snuck into a field of sweet clover and ate until they swelled up like balloons. Just in time, a farmer arrived and punctured the cows' stomachs with a knife, and the cows were saved. If the cows hadn't been stabbed, the fermentation gases from the clover would've remained trapped in their stomachs and they would've suffocated from the condition known as 'frothy bloat'. The illustration shows the cows rising shakily to their feet and being herded out of the deadly clover field. I remember that story because of the way it combined cruelty with mercy—the stabbing of the cows was the only way to save their lives. I remember agonising over this, because I couldn't stand the thought of hurting a cow or any animal. I have a half-theory that my ghost knife is fulfilling a similar function: when it stabs me, it releases something that's trapped. That thing is my anxiety. My personal frothy bloat. I feel a brief burst of relief, before inevitably I sneak into the sweet fields of worry again, gorging myself, the gas building up again, until I must be stabbed once more.

Intrusive thoughts can edge into much darker territory, especially when they become obsessive. If your thoughts become so preoccupying that they become debilitating, you likely have Obsessive Compulsive Disorder. Often reduced by pop culture to a cute and harmless quirk, OCD is popularly known as a condition whereby a person carries out repetitive behaviours such as checking, counting, tidying, praying; but it's the obsessive thoughts and uncertainties that compel those actions and which the sufferer is seeking to neutralise. Others have similarly obsessive thoughts but without the compulsions (or any that are observable), which is a lesser-known form of OCD: 'primarily obsessional OCD', or, colloquially, Pure O. With Pure O, the thoughts—always unwanted, sometimes violent, sexual, sacrilegious—are tortuous and difficult to articulate.

When reading some early accounts of what you could now call Pure O, it strikes me that nearly all of them describe thoughts that to their thinker were unmentionably blasphemous. In the seventh century, the monk Saint John Climacus wrote of an unholy demon that had a habit of showing up at church services and 'blaspheming the Lord and the consecrated elements'.[2] In 16th-century Germany, Martin Luther was reportedly haunted by images of the devil's bottom. Margery Kempe, medieval mystic and author of perhaps the first autobiography written in English, described her distress when she was unable to stop picturing men's penises—penises of all kinds, belonging to men 'both heathen and Christian, coming before her sight, so that she might not eschew them or put them out of her sight, showing their bare members unto her'. (Her book is written in the third person, as she dictated it to a priest.) 'It cannot be written what pain she felt and what sorrow she was in.'[3] Then there was Saint Ignatius of Loyola, founder of the Jesuit order, who lived in a little room which had a large hole in it. He would get so upset by the sins he thought he'd committed that he would have to restrain himself from throwing himself into the hole, the bottom of which he could not see.

Obsessive thoughts seem to run rings around deeply held beliefs. These thoughts are not 'benign or fairly neutral spontaneous mentation,' as one study puts it, 'but, rather, cognition with an "emotional bite".'[4] Contemporary accounts of Pure O are much more varied than the purely blasphemous; over the centuries, the places that people don't want their minds to go have branched and multiplied. People write of thoughts of harming their children, of throwing themselves out into traffic, of committing violent acts. 'A new friend and I were taking a walk in Marina del Rey on the bike path,' I read in a blog post

2   A.V. Avgoustidis, 'Obsessions from the Past: A Study of the Chapter on "Blasphemous Thoughts" in "The Ladder of Divine Ascent" (7th Century AD)', *Asian Journal of Psychiatry* 6, no. 6 (December 2013), 595–98.
3   Margery Kempe, *The Book of Margery Kempe: A Modern Version*, ed. W. Butler-Bowdon (London: Jonathan Cape, 1936), 352–3.
4   David A. Clark and Shelley Rhyno, 'Unwanted Intrusive Thoughts in Nonclinical Individuals: Implications for Clinical Disorders', in *Intrusive Thoughts in Clinical Disorders: Theory, Research, and Treatment*, ed. David A. Clark (Guilford Publications), 7.

by an OCD therapist. 'I asked her if she would like to walk to the jetty. I then had a thought: "When we get there I will kill you." I hope she doesn't read this blog!'[5]

My knife is a violent thought, and although its intensity ebbs and flows, I don't think it's consuming enough to take me into Pure O territory. Neither does it give rise to compulsive rituals or literal self-harm. It's a thought that leaves me feeling at best irritated and at worst bereft, but it turns up only once or twice a day, so perhaps it doesn't warrant treatment. Besides, some of the treatments sound, frankly, alarming. Exposure therapy is one. 'To combat the thought of hitting a pedestrian with a car, it started with me sitting in the driver's seat of the car and holding the wheel without the ignition on,' I read in one account of exposure therapy. 'Eventually, I got up to driving in a parking lot with a behavioral specialist running in front of the car.'

I try thinking about the knife directly to see if that lessens its power, as if thought itself could act as a shield. But this makes me even more preoccupied with the knife, and it becomes inventive in its shapeshifting, morphing into the tip of a scalding hot iron. I try to mock the knife and see it as ridiculous rather than disturbing: it's like a cartoon villain! He's wearing an invisibility cloak and sneaking up on me—cue suspenseful violins—but he's forgotten that everyone can see his giant knife! Then I worry that the ghost knife is somehow a phallic symbol and that I'm an even worse person than I'd thought, and this necessitates another stabbing.

Sometimes I just lie there staring into space, like Cletus the Slack-Jawed Yokel, thinking how weird it is that I can wring a sensation out of nothing. It's like rubbing your eyes and watching explosions unfurl under your eyelids, or seeing a thick woollen jumper on a bearded man and suddenly feeling itchy.

---

[5] Stacey Kuhl Wochner, 'Bizarre Thoughts and Me: Confessions of an OCD Therapist', *OCD Specialists* (blog), July 2013. ocdspecialists.com/bizarre-thoughts-and-me-confessions-of-an-ocd-therapist/

There must be an endless store of things you can feel, see, taste, if you happen to turn your mind in the right direction at the right time, like a butterfly net.

'So it comes out of the blue. This image of a knife pops into your mind and starts stabbing your face. And then: what do you think about that? What goes through your mind when that knife pops up?'

I'm in a session with my counsellor. To reassure me that I'm normal, she's just shown me a list from a landmark study in 1992 that names intrusive thoughts that are reportedly very common. Each of the thoughts is described as briefly as possible, as if the researcher wanted immediately to wash their hands of the matter. *Insulting authority figure. Breaking wind in public. Stabbing family member. Disgusting sex act. Cutting off finger. Fly undone.*[6] Well, if I hadn't already considered each of these acts, I have now.

I try to explain that while I don't feel good about the knife, I do feel a sort of relief each time it gets me. It's excruciating to listen back to my recording of the session, filled with lengthy pauses and my enthusiastic *Mmmm!* as the counsellor tries to help me clarify what it is I'm experiencing. (Climacus, again: 'It is extremely hard to articulate and to confess it and therefore to discuss it with a spiritual healer.') I tell her about my guilty and self-loathing thoughts before the knife appears, and I say, 'I think I probably *deserve* to be stabbed.'

My counsellor writes this down, murmuring, 'Think I probably deserve to be stabbed.' Then she says, 'People have all sorts of intrusions, and some of them can be quite weird and wonderful, eh? Now, if you were having this knife thought a lot more, and possibly undertaking a ritual as a result, that would

---

6   C. Purdon and D. Clark, 'Obsessive Intrusive Thoughts in Nonclinical Subjects: Part 1 Content and Relation with Depressive, Anxious and Obsessional Symptoms', *Behavior Research and Therapy* 31, no. 8 (1993): 713–20.

take us more into the realm of OCD, but you're not. The thing that's slightly different, here, perhaps, from common intrusive thoughts, is your *thinking* about the knife. You get stabbed, and you say to yourself, I deserved that.'

'Yes! And I never challenge it! I just think, "This is just the natural course of events for today."' It feels good to acknowledge what a pushover my brain is.

Although she doesn't offer any solutions, my counsellor does help me clarify the experience, in that way that simply saying something aloud can help you figure out what you're feeling. I have to acknowledge to myself, however, that as I get older, I am less and less satisfied by the answer 'what you are experiencing is very normal'. For one thing, I want to be told that I am special and unusual, and I want all mental health specialists to know this human weakness and indulge it. For another, knowing that what I am experiencing is normal makes me, stupidly, resent it more. For all its normality, why must it send us the signal that something is terribly wrong?

I wonder whether the thought of a knife is somewhat arbitrary—if it might be replaced, if I tried, by a feather, or a paintbrush, or a non-venomous snake. One OCD specialist whose blog I've been reading argues that the content of an intrusive thought doesn't actually matter. 'You will be equally tortured by any theme,' she says. 'As long as it's current, you decide it matters, and you are reactive to it.' So maybe it doesn't matter particularly that my thought is of a knife, but I'm *making it matter* by asking what's wrong with me. I already know that examining the thought closely or asking where it comes from only makes the knife more prominent, more autonomous. And when I go looking for it, there's plenty of evidence that this is indeed a thing—that attaching significance to an intrusive thought has a major bearing on how tightly it holds on. 'Greater attention and effort to control unwanted thoughts,' say intrusive thought researchers Clark and Rhyno, 'may actually lead to greater difficulty with the very thoughts one desires to avoid.'[7] This desperate need for avoidance, they say, causes the thinker to misattribute higher significance to the very thing they seek to minimise.

It seems that writing about the unwanted thought is the worst thing I could be doing. Well, I say to myself, that has never stopped me before.

I've read that a type of treatment called craniosacral therapy can help to 'relieve compression in the bones of the head', so I go to see a craniosacral therapist. The concept of craniosacral therapy sounds violent, but in practice it's barely even physical. The idea is that by very lightly holding the skull, the feet, and the back, the therapist can normalise the circulation of the fluid that surrounds the brain and spinal cord, removing 'blockages'. I describe my knife to the therapist and explain how tense it makes me feel. Maybe my knife is a blockage of some sort, I suggest, and maybe she can just, you know, remove it?

'Let's find out,' she says.

I lie down on the treatment table and the therapist takes my head into her hands. 'Some people feel a whooshing sensation as the cerebrospinal fluid flows upwards,' she says. I wait. Several fire trucks or ambulances blare past on the street outside. There is no whooshing sensation. The therapist holds my feet for a long time, with such a light pressure it's almost aggravating. It's like sitting at a table and wondering, Am I touching someone's foot, or is that a chair leg?

'I can hear your energy,' she is saying. At that point I lose interest completely and fall asleep.

More helpful than craniosacral therapy is watching a YouTube channel I've discovered called the ASMR Barber. The ASMR

---

[7] Clark and Rhyno, 11.

Barber, a gentle-looking bald-headed man—not actually a barber himself, as far as I can tell—travels around various countries, visiting barbershops along the way. He makes these videos, which are mostly very quiet but for distant noises of passing traffic, explicitly for the purpose of soothing the viewer. The ASMR Barber sits in the chair with his eyes closed as his head and face are sprayed with water, slathered in oil, and energetically rubbed to a shine. In one clip he visits a 'cosmic barber', whose signature head massage involves grabbing invisible, quick-moving things out of the air around the ASMR Barber's head. Somehow, watching someone else's head having attention lavished upon it has the effect of distancing me from my knife. At the end of one of these sessions, the ASMR Barber's head looks pure and bright, untouchable, almost eternal, like a star.

It's when I come across an essay by Matt Bieber, author of *Life in the Loop: Essays on OCD*, that I realise that there might be another way, albeit a harder way, of thinking about the knife, and thinking about what it's attacking. Bieber writes about how Buddhist teachings helped to subdue his intrusive thoughts; what specifically helped was accepting the Buddhist notion that there is no unified self at all. There is no core self to invade, nothing to unravel. Therefore, his various rituals—which he'd perceived as ways to keep himself unified, to counteract moments of confusion and disarray, to re-establish forward motion—are pointless. 'We are a kind of flux,' he writes, 'a series of patterns and surprises, inextricably interwoven into the larger field of phenomena that we call reality. Which means that we can't really let ourselves fall apart either, because we were never together in first place.'[8] This gives me the same vertiginous feeling I get when looking at a photograph of deep space. I don't know how to let go of my sense that my knife is attacking *me*—

8   Matt Bieber, 'Learning to Fall Apart', *Aeon*, 27 September 2013.

the self I recognise—and how to fathom the idea that I'm just a mass of things swirling around in space and the knife is swirling around amidst them all too, like a piece of space junk.

In her autobiography Margery Kempe referred to herself as 'this creature', which medieval scholars take to mean 'this creation of God'. She was known for expressing herself through loud cries, roars and sobs; she seemed to let every impulse flow through her. If it's true that we're in constant flux, with each momentary creation of ourselves giving way to another, maybe there's a way to let myself move more freely? Maybe the knife is just one more way that my brain is fighting to keep me, paradoxically, in one place and in one piece? 'The attempt to attain pleasure or avoid pain, to stay consistent with a storyline, to ensure some kind of outcome, to *be somebody*,' writes Bieber, 'this is what causes so much suffering.' Maybe I need to figure out a way to accept that I'm nobody, that I'm already in pieces. It almost seems too easy an answer, but it's also frightening. I think of John Lennon singing *relax and float downstream*, and wonder if the only way I'll know such freedom is through LSD or magic mushrooms or transcendental meditation, none of which are accessible to me right now.

I make a final appointment, this time with a psychiatrist. I've been putting this off, because seeing a psychiatrist is expensive. This whole investigation has been expensive. I would've been able to buy a whole bunch of literal knives by now if I hadn't been pursuing a solution to my ghost knife. As I sit in the psychiatrist's waiting room one weekday morning, along with a scattering of other women, I can see the privilege inherent in my situation. That I'm able to take an hour away from my job. That I'm able to pay to speak to a psychiatrist at all. That I'm able to write about this, even, without facing any particularly worrying social consequences.

The psychiatrist listens patiently as I stutter along—voicing this experience has become harder, not easier, through repetition, because I've come to expect that there won't be an answer—and then she offers a simple take. 'Your brain has figured out a way to commit emotional self-harm,' she says. 'Just like with cutting, you feel a small release, almost pleasure, when you think that thought. It provides a focus.'

There's something to this, I think. The knife's intent is unambiguous. It gives me something to resist—a situation to fight, a story I don't want to be true. But it also provides a release. I think of the cows in the field of clover again.

A friend tells me about a time when he'd just had his ears syringed, and later was walking home at night. Along the way he began to feel spooked because he could hear a strange sound. 'I felt convinced I was being followed,' he said. Later, he realised: 'It was the sound of my own trousers.' This is the most accurate descriptor of generalised anxiety I've come across: the sound of your own trousers. With my generalised anxiety ('You are haunted by persistent sensations of discomfort running through all the levels of your being', one recent self-test tells me; I can't help but imagine this sentence being hollered from a passing car), I can't usually pinpoint what it is that causes the dread and chaos I sometimes feel; though in a quieter moment I'll realise I was just lonely. I try to ward the feeling off through intense exercise, medication, and, too often, isolating myself, as I long for containment and safety.

When I get home that night, I try something: I just hold my head in my hands and rub the side of my face for a long time, the muscles that feel sore and knotted from tensing. My cat watches me intently, probably wondering why I'm not stroking him instead. I am going to keep trying to solve my ghost knife; I want to burrow underneath it and prise it out forever. But in this moment, holding my head helps. This gentleness provides a different focus. It helps just to hold my head, feeling its weird, soft, whole fullness.

Mountain View Road

Mikey Dam

Reach inside my thoughts
And figure out my happiness
Because anxiety
Had really got me trapped in this

I had my first panic attack on Cuba Street in Palmerston North. I was hyperventilating and short of breath, and I didn't know what was happening. I was too afraid to see a doctor.

At the time, I was with a girl who I'd been seeing for three years. She was someone I was close to, and so comfortable being around, but I kept the panic inside. I remember sitting in cafes with her and finding it hard to breathe, not understanding what was wrong with me. I never told her, or anyone, what I was experiencing, and I tried to ignore it.

But the panic attacks kept coming, and I couldn't stop them. At night, I was afraid to sleep, scared I'd never wake up. Nighttime was too quiet. Regret, thoughts and memories would pop up and my brain wouldn't stop working. I thought about how, a few years prior, I had been in and out of schools and been in trouble with the police; I was just repeating mistakes. Now I was regretting a lot of my choices. I was always asking 'Why? What makes me think this way?' It was a question I couldn't answer. I hated the night-time.

I was too young to apply for the benefit, so I enrolled in a course so that I could get money from StudyLink. But I had no guidance around what to do with my life, and I couldn't handle it anymore. I felt broken. My relationship with my girlfriend was failing because I had no job and I was terrible with money. I was drinking a lot. I thought alcohol would help me stay happy and comfortable. I would drink on nights where I had course the next day; I didn't care what anybody thought about me for those few hours I was intoxicated. I was lost.

I felt like everyone had given up on me, and I didn't know where I was headed. Depression caught up with me from the hangovers and the constant regret, and I still hadn't talked to anybody about it. It had been five months I'd spent in this dark place that I still didn't have a name for. I had stomach problems caused by the anxiety I was feeling. One day I just knew I had had enough, and I broke down. I called my mum.

I rarely talk to my mum, but I trusted her. We met at Subway for dinner and I had a little bit of money that I offered to use to pay for hers. But she wouldn't let me pay. She knew I wasn't really financially stable, or, as I would say, balling. We got to eating and she asked me, 'What's up?'

I had planned this conversation all week, and knowing that I was about to tell her I was depressed and anxious made me feel weak and stupid. But I knew I needed help. I explained everything, and my mum was shocked. She told me to move home.

Being at my mum's helped me feel stable, so I had time to make music. I had always enjoyed making music as a hobby, but I didn't realise then that I was going to chase music as a career—and nor did I realise it would save my life.

Even while making music I was still having day-to-day problems. I was so bad when it came to talking with people about how I felt emotionally—I just wouldn't let anybody know, not even my family. Instead, I put all of my thoughts into my music. I wrote about my life, about things that held me down for years. The music was letting me speak.

Over time I start to progress in music, and it started to become more fluent. I began to work with the Noble brothers, who were long-time family friends. When people complimented me on my music, it made me realise I was doing something with my life. Self-fulfilment wasn't something I'd understood before—all my life, I'd just wanted to make everybody proud of me. Up until then I'd been making music to make me feel as though I was doing something with myself, but now I was starting to feel proud of myself, and proud of my music in its own right.

In Palmerston North, I went a few years without feeling anxiety and having panic attacks. I had done a lot of searching for answers that helped clear the air with a few people I was close with. My partner and I broke up and I bounced in out of houses couch-surfing, but the music kept me feeling like I had someone to talk to. Over time I gained knowledge of my craft, and with the Nobles producing, I started to turn what we were doing for fun into a career. I wanted to be someone to people, but I also wanted to hold on to this way of speaking my mind when I couldn't do that with words. What was a hobby now became everything I wanted in life.

In September 2017 I got a call from an uncle who asked if I wanted to move to Auckland. By this time music was flowing and opening doors of opportunity and I thought that the biggest leap of my career was about to begin. I was a small-city kid who wanted more in life than a 9 to 5 job. I decided to make the move to Auckland.

A few days before flying, I got restless. I couldn't sleep and I had chest pains and a sore stomach. I realised I was afraid of moving. I was comfortable where I was in Palmerston North: I had a great family and an amazing girlfriend who supported me, and I knew deep down I wanted to stay—but I also wanted to pursue my dream. I called a friend. 'You're just nervous, bro,' he told me. 'This will benefit your career. Take the leap—you've got nothing to lose.' I thought, He's right. If I don't like it I'll come back.

Auckland was an amazing place. A massive eye-opener, full of opportunity and hustle. But I was working a job that I hated, where there was a lot of drug use and I was talked down to. My anxiety got heavy three weeks in. I started to realise how much I missed home and couldn't wrap my head around why I was having these anxiety attacks. Although I'm Māori, my skin is light. I was working with people who had darker skin than me, and they thought I was Pākehā. I felt separate from them even though they had the same skin colour as my nan and my father. My upbringing was apparently better than others. I felt alone and silenced by everyone. 'Go home to the North Shore,' they'd say. 'You're white.'

I became scared to sleep again. Scared to go out and eat. Scared to go to work. I didn't like being in a studio with artists I barely knew; I didn't want to meet new people—I just wanted to stay by myself and write. Anywhere I went in Auckland, I felt anxious—it was the worst it had ever been. Nothing I did was good enough. I felt as though I was always trying to open a door, but every time I took a step forward the door moved forward too. At the same time, the more I wrote, the better I felt inside about my direction in music.

At Christmas that year, I went home to spend the holiday with my family. I thought being around them would make me comfortable and relaxed, but it didn't. I felt paranoid and I was constantly thinking about going back to Auckland. Why didn't I just go back? Auckland could be my ticket to success, and I was gonna stick it out. I didn't want to accept failure. But I began to put my dreams before my health.

I went back to the city in the New Year. As soon as I went back, my panic attacks grew worse. My anxiety was hitting me hard at work, and I was being talked to like a kid who knew nothing. I felt trapped in an ugly place. Deep down I wanted to die, but I didn't want people to think I had given up so I fought through those suicidal feelings. When I was told my dreams were far-fetched and that it was impossible to be as big as the people I looked up to, I started to believe it.

One night, lying in bed, I watched a YouTube video of myself performing in 2009. I looked so happy. I went through old photos, trying to remember what I'd been doing that day, trying to figure out why I had been so uncomplicatedly happy. I just wanted to be that guy again. After watching that video I stayed up all night, too afraid to sleep. I had sharp pains in my chest and automatically thought the worst.

When I woke up the next morning after two hours' sleep, my partner called and asked if I was okay. I started crying. I was shattered. I didn't want to give up on my dreams of being a successful musician but I knew the time was coming to get myself right. That night, my friend, one of the Noble brothers, was coming to Auckland. I decided to catch a ride back with him. I packed my bags and I went home to Palmerston North the next day.

It was so good to know I was going home. This time I would make sure I sorted myself out for good. I found myself in a place of comfort, writing music at odd times and in weird places. I listened to songs that reminded me of places where I'd been happy, songs my nan would play me as a kid, like Delegation's 'Oh Honey'. I felt like I was moving closer to myself, back to who I was.

After a while, I went to the doctor and was diagnosed with clinical depression, and prescribed antidepressants. Being around my family and my partner and spending time in places where I felt comfortable helped me to relax, and I started to feel that I could be more open about what I had been through. As soon as I started talking about it, I felt a massive weight lift from my shoulders. I continued to speak up about my anxiety, and along the way people talked to me about what they were going through too. I started to feel normal. I started to feel a part of something.

In April 2018, I went on *Native Affairs* and revealed that I suffered from anxiety. I released my single about depression and anxiety, 'Mountain View Road', not long after. Mountain View Road in Palmerston North is one of the places I would go to clear my thoughts when I was feeling overwhelmed, and the song is about everything that makes me happy, as well as everything that causes my anxiety. It is one of the truest stories I've ever written, and in three weeks, it reached 100,000 streams on Spotify.

It was writing music that got me through. I still feel anxious sometimes—not as much as before, and it is manageable now. I'd started making music because I was in love with writing my life and sharing my stories with the world. When I write, I portray my life with honesty, and my music is a reflection of how I feel. That's what I hope people will hear when they listen to my work.

As Fresh as They Come

Tusiata Avia

I usually know what I'm writing about, but this time I don't. I am stumbling about half blind. I'm writing this to try to figure out what's happening to me. It's been about six weeks since I've become aware that I have anxiety and depression. I'm about as fresh as they come.

I'm struggling through a place which is in one way familiar to me, but which has become so intense that everything seems strange, warped, weirdly mirrored, morphing—a funhouse without the fun. And I am the strangest thing of all. Am I dying? What is really wrong with me? Why have I been sick for so long? Will I ever get better? This is the current, constant loop of my thinking.

The human intestines are said to be kilometres long, twisting and turning around and around upon themselves. They are like my thoughts. I am sick in them. I have been for a year. My thoughts coil around and around. I float outside the skin of my stomach imagining my insides, and worrying.

Yesterday, I was talking with a close friend, and our conversation made me aware how very new this territory is to me, even though in some ways I've lived here for years without realising or being able to name it. Till now, I've been able to tough it out.

My friend—who I have taken to calling Sensei H for her hard-won wisdom—says anxiety is free-wheeling. It roams the landscape and will latch on to anything that's there. That is its nature, she says. Yes! I want to shout, because after a year of pain, fatigue, fainting and now depression and anxiety—which a specialist recently told me are all symptoms of problems in my gut—I have become anxious about my stomach. Leave me by myself for five minutes, and I'll start obsessing about it.

A number of weeks ago, before my visit to the specialist, it was my parenting I felt anxious about. This was when Uso, another wonderful friend, sat me down and said, 'You are depressed.' It was like a slap in the face. It woke me up. The next day I was at the doctor and she was prescribing me Citalopram.

I've never really believed in antidepressants—not for myself, that is. For other people—sure, fine; some kind of chemical imbalance, absolutely. But, for me, antidepressants are tightly connected with a sense of failure. And if I feel I have failed, I feel shame.

Shame is a dark dancing partner and he prefers—he demands—complete silence. Sewn-up lips. I believe Shame must be unmasked, brought into the centre of the room; the hypnotic music must be turned off and the lights turned on. For me, this is the remedy that dissolves the stitches and stops the dreadful tango. Yes, it's scary to out myself to the world. That's what I'm doing in this essay. I could continue to be the Facebook version of Tusiata: Look at her at this festival, at that play, at this reading—looking fabulous. But the 40 kilograms I've lost in the last year is because my gut is sick, and in a couple of hours I will pass out on the bathroom floor. And then when I get home from the fabulous festival to Aranui, I'll be Tusiata in her dressing gown. This Tusiata is struggling with depression, anxiety, fatigue and pain. This Tusiata is unable to eat. She is all the things no one takes selfies of.

While researching my symptoms to try to understand what was happening to me, I came across a book called *Gut* by Giulia Enders. Enders talks about the incredibly close links between gut health and brain health. I've found myself and my symptoms exactly described in her book. One thing that sticks in my mind is the fact that 95 percent of the serotonin (the 'happy chemical') produced by a person is manufactured in the cells of the gut.

So it makes sense that someone who suffers from anxiety or depression might also have an unhappy gut. 'We should not always blame depression on the brain or on our life circumstances,' writes Enders. 'There is much more to us than that.'

Medication has helped me to deal with the at times unbearable stress of being a single working mother. This stress is something I've suffered with ever since I became one. My stress levels would get so intense I would have to lock myself in my bedroom to keep both my child and myself safe. With medication, that changed. Suddenly, enough space opened up inside me that I wasn't down to the wire with my parenting *all* the time. Now when there is stress with my child—which is most of the time—I have something to go on. I have some room, some give, some perspective. The feeling of being able to *cope* with this stress is an absolute revelation to me. After more than a decade of feeling like a monstrously flawed parent and human being, it has given me relief.

My anxiety has not been so easily 'fixed' by medication. I felt a decrease in the anxiety for a while—perhaps while the medication first kicked in—but in the last week I've noticed it ramp up again. I think I knew during that first month of medication, through that slightly drugged feeling, that the anxiety was still there, only suppressed. Now it's back. My thoughts loop back again and again to my stomach, of course, and to my work, around which I feel paralysed. Those are the two biggest at the moment: my gut, and my work.

Sensei H said that in her 20s and 30s she was afraid of chairs. She was afraid that if she sat down she wouldn't be able to get up again. Yes! I almost shouted in recognition. The paralysis! I realise I've had some measure of this since I was about 15 years old. Now the dial on the paralysis seems to be stuck up on high most of time. In its wake comes anxiety, because I feel I haven't achieved enough.

Like my school reports: *Tusiata needs to work harder.* I've always thought that working harder was the panacea to my problems. But it's not. It really, really is not. That is the voice of anxiety. Even I can recognise that. Anxiety with its cat-o-nine tails thrashing me onwards towards more anxiety.

Perfectionism is something that perhaps makes me a good poet. The drafting and redrafting, the obsessive over and over, down to the word, the letter, the punctuation mark. Perfectionism works for a poem; it doesn't work for so many other things. In fact, I've got to be careful I don't get all perfectionist with this essay! Perfectionism can be a disease; it folds in on itself; with its origami teeth it eats you up. Nothing is ever good enough; you're not good enough. Outside of poetry, perfectionism has not served me. Perfectionism has been anxiety masquerading. It has driven me to work far too hard. For fear. It has allowed other people to take advantage of me and work me far too hard. It has caused me enormous stress. It has been part of the frightening funhouse carousel of the breakdown of my health.

My dear friend Uso has also been on Citalopram and has been an invaluable help to me as I navigate the depression, anxiety and the drug itself. When I had the sudden and frightening return of anxiety, and a particularly dark weekend, Uso reassured me that I wasn't crashing back into depression but was probably coming to some kind of baseline after 5–6 weeks on the drug. This, Uso said, was the time to notice that I still had the space to think about what was good for me (they were right; I did by the Monday) and make the small plans and adjustments to life so I felt better. Uso made the important point that it was also about doing the mahi myself, not just using the meds only. This for me means getting regular exercise, connecting with people, finding a counsellor and writing. Writing this essay is part of it.

As a writer, I usually have a clever way to bring a piece

of writing to a close—an elegant, strong, poetic ending. But writing this piece has been like groping through a strange twilit terrain. I'm tottering around with a small flickering torch and I can only make out small patches here and there. I have yet to find a vantage point from which I can see the full sweep of this land I'm in. I guess after six weeks it's probably expecting a bit much of myself.

I've been extremely fortunate to have a couple of experienced, well-travelled, wise guides who know the lay of the land, who remember how things work in this country and have been able to report back from the frontlines. This has made a huge difference. So, too, have a number of kind friends. At this point I can offer you this essay as my own sputtering flashlight as I stumble about in these early days, trying to find my feet, and I hope that this—or one of the other essays in this book—helps.

Contributors

TUSIATA AVIA was born in Christchurch in 1966 and is of Samoan and Palagi descent. She is an acclaimed poet, performer and children's book writer. Her poetry collections include *Fale Aitu | Spirit House* (VUP, 2016), *Wild Dogs Under My Skirt* (VUP, 2004; also staged as a one-woman theatre show around the world from 2002–08) and *Bloodclot* (VUP, 2009). Tusiata has held the Fulbright Pacific Writer's Fellowship at the University of Hawai'i in 2005 and the Ursula Bethell Writer in Residence at University of Canterbury in 2010. She was the 2013 recipient of the Janet Frame Literary Trust Award.

HINEMOANA BAKER is a poet, musician, occasional broadcaster and creative writing teacher. She traces her mixed ancestry from several Māori tribes, as well as from England and Bavaria. Her first book, *matuhi | needle*, was co-published in 2004 by Victoria University Press and actor Viggo Mortensen's Perceval Press. Since then, she has published two more poetry collections (VUP, 2010, 2014) and has edited several more anthologies. She has produced and released several albums of original music, as well as a CD of field recordings and text gathered while she lived in Australia. Her work pivots around sonic art, lyric, experimental poetry and family storytelling. She works in English, Māori and more recently German, the latter in collaboration with German poet and sound performer Ulrike Almut-Sandig. She is currently living in Berlin, where she was 2016 Creative New Zealand Berlin Writer in Residence.

MEREDITH BLAMPIED is a registered clinical psychologist and PhD student in the Mental Health and Nutrition Research Group. She gained her postgraduate diploma in clinical psychology from the University of Canterbury. She works predominantly with adults experiencing severe anxiety disorders. Meredith's research interests include the role of nutrition in mental health and she explores feedback-informed treatment and best-evidence practice for anxiety disorders, particularly obsessive compulsive disorder. She is involved in ongoing research on the impact of the Canterbury earthquakes on an anxious population.

AIMIE CRONIN is an award-winning freelance journalist who writes about human interest and social justice issues for the *NZ Listener*, *NZ Herald*, *Metro* and other publications. She is based in Hamilton and is currently a stay-at-home mum with her baby boy.

MIKEY DAM (Michael Luke) is a 24-year-old songwriter and recording artist with Universal Music and Sony Music NZ. His debut mixtape in 2017, *MNO*, received top ratings from popular music blogs and magazines internationally. He has since gone on to release another chart-topping single, 'Mountain View Road'. He grew up surrounded by music in Manaia and now lives in Auckland, where he produces singles for New Zealand's top artists.

ALLAN DREW has a PhD in English and Creative Writing from Victoria University of Wellington. His PhD project involved writing a novel that fictionalised the life of John Milton while he was writing *Paradise Lost*. Allan's short stories, non-fiction and poems have appeared in publications across New Zealand, Australia, the UK and US. He is a fiction reader for *Overland* and teaches Creative Writing and Science Communication at Massey University.

BONNIE ETHERINGTON's novel *The Earth Cries Out* (Vintage NZ, 2017) was shortlisted for the 2018 William Saroyan International Prize for Writing and longlisted for the Ockham New Zealand Book Awards. She has a Master's in Creative Writing from Massey University, and her short fiction, poetry and nonfiction have appeared in publications including *Guernica, Landfall, Headland, Ika, Meniscus* and *Takahē*. She was born in Nelson, raised in West Papua, and currently lives in Chicago with her husband and cat while she works towards a PhD in Literature at Northwestern University.

D.A. GLYNN was born and raised on Auckland's North Shore. He worked in pre-press, design and copywriting for 15 years. He has lived in Auckland, San Francisco, London and Sydney. He has published three books of non-fiction—on chefs, salt and bestselling authors—and one novel. He plays guitar, bass, drums and piano. For the last few years he has been largely nomadic, but right now he lives in Dunedin, where he plays bass for Jay Clarkson & the Containers and cooks chilli at the Inch Bar on Tuesdays.

RIKI GOOCH (Ngai Tāhūhū / Patuharakeke) is an award-winning composer, producer, sound artist and multi-instrumentalist based in Wellington. *He hono tāngata e kore e motu; kāpā he taura waka e motu.* Unlike a rope; a human bond can never be severed.

PAULA HARRIS was the 2017 recipient of the Lilian Ida Smith Award. Her work has appeared in *The Spinoff, Poetry NZ Yearbook, Snorkel, Landfall, Takahē* and *Broadsheet*. She sleeps a lot, because that's what depression makes you do. Paula was born in Palmerston North in 1973.

KATE KENNEDY is a 51-year-old author, musician and registered nurse. She currently works in the tourism sector. In 2011 she published a memoir, *Matters To A Head: Cannabis, Mental Illness and Recovery*, about her 15-year battle to overcome cannabis addiction while living with bipolar disorder. Born in Motueka, she is a nomad and is at present based in Marlborough with her wife, pets and a family of eels.

MICHELLE LANGSTONE is a writer and actor. She has written about literature and art for the *NZ Listener*, *The Pantograph Punch* and *Newsroom*. Her acting work includes *800 Words*, *The Almighty Johnsons* and *McLeod's Daughters*. She divides her time between Sydney and Auckland.

ROSEMARY MANNERING has been working as a registered physiotherapist since 1963. She became interested in treating mental health after being offered a job as a physiotherapist in the Christchurch Mental Health Facility (then called Sunnyside Hospital). In 1994 she was awarded a Winston Churchill Fellowship and visited Britain to study the role of physiotherapy in mental health. In 2000 she established StressCare Physiotherapy in Christchurch, specialising in techniques to help ease stress, anxiety and insomnia, correct hyperventilation, and manage chronic pain. Rosemary has presented at conferences for the New Zealand Society of Physiotherapists, run postgraduate courses for physiotherapists and taught undergraduate students on the links between mental health and the body.

EAMONN MARRA is a comedian, writer and zine-maker who lives in Wellington. He's best known for his comedy about anxiety and mental illness. He has performed in the New Zealand International Comedy Festival and the New Zealand Fringe Festival, and has appeared on TV3's AotearoHA Rising Stars. He is one of the hosts of the storytelling podcast *What We Talk About*. His writing has appeared in *Sport*, *The Spinoff*, and *The Wireless*.

SELINA TUSITALA MARSH, celebrated poet and scholar, is the first Pasifika Poet Laureate in New Zealand (2018–20). Of Samoan, Tuvaluan, English, Scottish and French descent, Tusitala Marsh was the first PI to graduate with a PhD in English from the University of Auckland, where she's now an associate professor lecturing in creative writing and Pacific literature. Her poetry collections include *Fast Talking PI* (AUP, 2009), which won the 2010 NZSA Jessie Mackay Best First Book Award for Poetry, *Dark Sparring* (AUP, 2013) and *Tightrope* (AUP, 2017). Her work has been published in over 70 national and international anthologies, academic books, literary and scholarly journals and on various notable literary websites. In 2017 she was editor of *Best New Zealand Poems*.

JESS McALLEN is a Wellington-based freelance journalist who writes about social issues and health. Her work has appeared in (among other publications) *NZ Geographic*, *Mana*, the *NZ Listener*, *The Spinoff*, *Radio New Zealand* and *Sunday*.

KIRSTEN McDOUGALL is the author of two works of fiction, *The Invisible Rider* (VUP, 2012) and *Tess* (VUP, 2017). She was the recipient of the 2013 Creative New Zealand Louis Johnson New Writer's Bursary, and won the short category of 'The Long and the Short of It' fiction competition in 2011. *Tess* was longlisted for the 2018 Ockham New Zealand Book Awards and shortlisted for the 2018 Ngaio Marsh Awards.

DANYL McLAUCHLAN was born in Wellington in 1974. He studied at Victoria University of Wellington and worked and travelled in Europe, the Middle East and Asia before he returned to Wellington, where he works as a biologist. He is the author of the comic noir novels *Unspeakable Secrets of the Aro Valley* (VUP, 2013) and *Mysterious Mysteries of the Aro Valley* (VUP, 2016).

DONNA McLEOD lives in Motueka surrounded by whānau on McLeod Bennett Papakaiinga in the rohe of Te Āti Awa and Ngāti Rārua and Te Āwhina Marae. Born in Taranaki, she is a child of Parihaka and Muru Raupatu. She is a writer and performer of Te Ora Haa and a member of Te Ohu Whakaari.

LEE MURRAY is a ten-time winner of New Zealand's Sir Julius Vogel Award for science fiction, fantasy, and horror. Her titles include the bestselling military thriller *Into the Mist* and supernatural crime-noir *Hounds of the Underworld* (co-authored with Dan Rabarts), both of which were longlisted for the international Bram Stoker® Award. She is proud to have co-edited nine anthologies, including one which won her an Australian Shadows Award in 2014. She lives with her family in the sunny Bay of Plenty.

REBECCA PRIESTLEY is an award-winning science writer and historian. Her essay 'Lucky to Be Here' is from her forthcoming book with VUP, published 2019. She is the author of the acclaimed *Mad on Radium: New Zealand in the Atomic Age* (AUP, 2012) and the editor of several major anthologies, the latest of which is *Dispatches from Continent Seven: An Anthology of Antarctic Science* (Awa Press, 2016). Rebecca is associate professor at the Science in Society Group at Victoria University of Wellington, and in 2016 she won the Prime Minister's Science Communication Prize. In 2018 she was made a Companion by the Royal Society Te Apārangi.

MADELINE REID is a writer, musician and teacher. She has an MA in Creative Writing from the International Institute of Modern Letters and her work has been published in *Landfall*, *Mimicry*, *Turbine*, *Aotearotica* and *The Wireless*. She lives and works in Auckland.

JULIA RUCKLIDGE is a professor of clinical psychology at the Department of Psychology and the director of the Mental Health and Nutrition Research Group. Originally from Toronto, she completed her PhD at the University of Calgary in clinical psychology followed by a postdoctoral fellowship at the Hospital for Sick Children in Toronto. In the last decade, she and her lab have been running clinical trials investigating the role of broad-spectrum micronutrients in the expression of mental illness. In 2015 Julia was the recipient of the Ballin Award from the NZ Psychologist Society and was also named one of the 100 Most Influential Women in New Zealand. In 2018 she received a Braveheart award for her contribution to making Christchurch a better place to live.

SUSAN STRONGMAN is an Auckland-based journalist at *The Wireless*. She likes to spend her spare time with her cats.

KERRY SUNDERLAND is Nelson Arts Festival Readers and Writers programme coordinator and a part-time creative writing tutor at Nelson Marlborough Institute of Technology. She is a writer, freelance journalist, magazine editor, film reviewer and radio presenter/producer. Kerry was awarded a Master of Arts in Creative Writing from the International Institute of Modern Letters at Victoria University of Wellington in 2017 and, after being offered the Hachette Mentorship for 2018, hopes she is in the final stages of preparing her memoir, *Beyond the Blue Door*, for publication.

ZION TAUAMITI is a mentor for young men at Christchurch-based Bros For Change, developed by former New Zealand Māori and New Zealand Rugby League player Jaye Pukepuke. Before that, he worked as a life promotion worker with non-profit health and social service organisation He Waka Tapu, visiting around 12 schools a week and supporting thousands of young people. He is also a musician, weaver, and founder of community choir the Pou Tiriao Singers. He ran for the Māori Party for Christchurch East in the last election.

HOLLY WALKER is a writer and book reviewer based in Lower Hutt. She served as a Green MP from 2011–14, before stepping down after having her first child. Her reviews and essays have appeared in *The Spinoff*, *The Wireless*, *Sunday* and *Your Weekend*, and in several edited collections. Her short memoir *The Whole*

Intimate Mess: Motherhood, Politics, and Women's Writing was published by Bridget Williams Books in 2016. She is now based at home, caring for her two daughters and working on her PhD in creative writing at the International Institute of Modern Letters.

YVETTE WALKER is an Australian writer living in New Zealand. Her debut novel *Letters to the End of Love* (UQP) won a 2014 WA Premier's Book Award and was also shortlisted for a NSW Premier's Book Award. She is currently working full-time on her second book.

PAUL STANLEY WARD is a Wellington writer and producer. After gaining a master's degree at Oxford and producing for a Discovery Channel show, he returned home and wrote for television documentary series *Here to Stay* and *Undercover*. He received a Qantas Best Screenplay Award for the short film *The Graffiti of Mr Tupaia* (2008) and co-produced the award-winning website *Wild Eyes* and kids' TV spinoff *Wild Peeps*. Paul was founding editor of the screen showcase website *NZ On Screen*. The lifelong bird nerd leads the conservation projects Polhill Protectors and Capital Kiwi. His writing has appeared in the *NZ Listener*, *Forest & Bird*, *The Spinoff*, *Atlas* and *UpCountry*.

SARAH LIN WILSON is a writer from Nelson. Her work has appeared in *New Zealand Geographic*, *The Wireless* and *Sport*. Her hobbies include late-night online shopping, pretending she doesn't have any unread emails and using too many em-dashes.

ASHLEIGH YOUNG is an editor at Victoria University Press. She is the author of the poetry collection *Magnificent Moon* (VUP, 2012) and the essay collection *Can You Tolerate This?* (VUP, 2016). An abridged version of her essay 'Ghost Knife' has appeared on *The Cut* (New York Media).